At Home Delivery

Dad's Story

At Home Delivery

Dad's Story

Kennedy Wolf

Copyright Page

Published in: Grand Island, Florida USA
By: LakeHill Publishing Inc
Requests for permissions should be forwarded to:
info@lakehillpublishing.com

First Edition
Author: **Kennedy Wolf**
At Home Delivery - Dad's Story
Designed By: LakeHill Publishing Inc
ISBN: 979-8-88582-012-7 Softcover
ISBN: 979-8-88582-013-4 Hardcover
ISBN: 979-8-88582-014-1 Digital
Printed In the United States of America

Disclaimer

At Home Delivery, Dad's Story: is one man's story of Nonfiction. Names, dates and regions have been changed to protect the privacy of individuals spoken of in this book. Some of the stories in this book are pretty graphic and personal reader discretion is advised! This book was written for adults and not intended for children to read. This book is not a replacement for medical advice.

This book offers the events and opinions of the author and his family. The stories written in this book were actual events and the author does not endorse that you recreate any of the events that he or his family have experienced throughout the birthing process, without being under the care of licensed professionals. The information stated in this book should not be used as a substitute for a care provider, and in no way is the author offering any Medical or Care advice to anyone for any reason. Any act or action written in this book was performed while under the care of licensed medical professionals, please seek assistance from your medical provider if you are ever in a similar situation.

The publisher and the author are providing this book and its contents on an "as is" basis and make no representations or warranties of any kind with respect to this book or its contents. The publisher and the author disclaim all such representations and warranties, including but not limited to warranties of healthcare for a particular purpose. In addition, the publisher and the author assume no responsibility for errors, inaccuracies, omissions, or any other inconsistencies herein.

The content of this book is for informational purposes only and is not intended to diagnose, treat, cure, or prevent any condition or disease. You understand that this book is not intended as a substitute for consultation with a licensed practitioner. Please consult with your own physician or healthcare specialist regarding the suggestions and recommendations made in this book. The use of this book implies your acceptance of this disclaimer.

The publisher and the author make no guarantees concerning the level of success you may experience by following the stories or strategies contained in this book, and you accept the risk that results will differ for each individual. The testimonials and examples provided in this book show exceptional results, which may not apply to the average reader, and are not intended to represent or guarantee that you will achieve the same or similar results. Reader discretion is advised.

Dedication

This book was written for Emily.
Thank you for giving me my son!

Kennedy

Table of Contents

Introduction

The choices we make tend to follow us throughout our day-to-day life. Is one person's story better than another? I don't believe it is. Everyone has a story to tell. Life is made up of events that take place, to leave timestamps in your memory. These events can be stored up until they are told at a later date. Well, that later date for me is today.

The best way for me to tell you my story is with two different birthing experiences I lived. The perfect pregnancy and delivery is the one that I just experienced. The less-than-ideal pregnancy and delivery was one that I experienced 17 years ago, when my daughter was born.

I am in no way an expert at pregnancy, delivery or birth. My point of view is all that I have to offer. Seeing as I have been through a less than ideal pregnancy and now an almost perfect one, I would like to get it off my chest. The story you are about to read is my story. The events happened to myself and my family. These were the actual events that took place. They are not made up in any way.

It's my hope that my story will help someone when they need this help the most. I apologize in advance for any misspellings or grammatical errors in this book, I am a farmer not an editor. Like I said, these are my words.

Chapter 1

Dad's Story

The thought of being a dad for the first time was pretty big news to me. Finding out that you're going to be a dad for the second time is pretty exhilarating. Fatherhood is not something to take for granted, and it can break down even the toughest of men. I mean that in a great way. It will make you more sensitive to the way you now view your life. The dad title also makes you a bigger protector over your family as well. Now you will do anything you can to keep them safe.

Trying to explain how great it was to welcome my daughter into this world is hard to do. The fact is, yes, she was healthy and beautiful. Unfortunately, the first time I was able to meet her, was in the waiting room at a hospital. A waiting room that was just a short walk down the hall from the operating room. This was my new residence, as she was surgically removed by a scalpel and hospital staff that I never even had the opportunity to meet.

I was not invited in to see the birth of my daughter, nor would the hospital allow me to look through the door. Instead, I sat in an empty waiting room with several chairs and a door that was shut off from the hallway. There was dead silence. When someone would walk by, I would get up and open the door to see if they had my child for me to see.

Honestly, I'm a pretty tough man. I can hit my finger with a hammer while nailing up a fence, and not shed a tear. On this day however, I couldn't control my emotions, I was letting it all out. The collar of my shirt was soaking wet from where I was wiping my tears.

The thoughts running through my head were filling the emptiness of the room. I didn't have a smart phone to play music, or even a television to watch to help pass the time. All that I had were my thoughts, and they were not the most positive.

When you are put in a situation that you didn't sign up for, it can change the way that you think. I had no one to call, as everyone I knew couldn't answer their telephones. The cell service in this hospital was nonexistent anyway. I was alone, I just wanted things to be normal again.

After going through, what I would consider, one of the tougher parts of my life. The things that made them tough were now in the past. I had an open mind and a free heart. Putting that experience in the past I was now ready to move on and Clare, my daughter's mother, has moved on as well.

A lot of years have passed by now, along with several long-term relationships that I put behind me. I would say that my first experience of having a child, deterred me from wanting another. This led to my daughter growing up without siblings. The scars that I had from the first experience made me not want to try again.

I have heard it said that time heals everything! Well, I can say that time heals a lot of things, but not everything. The time isn't the factor in my case, it was being able to open my heart again and let goodness in.

Meeting the love of my life seemed to be a gift that was sent to me for all the hard work that I put in over the years. Just a few years ago when I was losing my path in life, I asked for the perfect person to come into my life and make me happy again. It took a little time and then my wish did come true.

They say when you meet *the one* you will just know. Well let me tell you, I didn't think that Emily was the one at first! I kept telling myself that she couldn't be the one. She was a lot younger than me and she was quite mysterious. I wasn't really into solving puzzles, so I wasn't sure that I could make her mine.

When we bumped into each other the first time, she was with an older man! That was intriguing to me, as I am an older man, but I'm in no way a homewrecker. Before we parted ways from the small chat we had, I told her who I was and where my farm was located. She was equally intrigued with me now. At least I thought she was by the smile on her face. I offered that if she ever needed anything to just let me know and I gave her my phone number.

Turns out that the older man she was with wasn't her husband or her boyfriend after all. That man was her *dad*! She made sure to make that fact well known, that evening, when she clarified it over a text message to me. She stated she was single and not looking to be locked down anytime soon.

Now the wheels in my head were turning. What are the odds that I would meet this woman on the night before we were forecasted to have a hurricane hit landfall in our area? I was thinking that fate may have brought us to meet each other. Or there could be another reason that I'm not sure about. Only thing that matters is that Emily is now my wife and the mother to my newborn baby boy.

Emily and I thought that we had planned for every scenario possible. While we did a great job being ready for the baby to finally be in our arms, we might have missed a few things that would have made the birthing process a lot easier. Being forgetful is not a crime, there are things that come up while you are under pressure that you forget about. There are situations that you never figured you would be dealing with.

I hope that my story will help someone when they need the help the most.

Chapter 2

Pre-Pregnancy

Emily and I were married, with the understanding, that we really didn't want to have children of our own. I already had my daughter from a previous relationship and she was perfectly fine with that.

Emily had this dream of putting her 4-year college degree to work. Climbing the ranks at the Fortune 500 company she worked for. We were living a comfortable life. I would go to work daily as a logistics manager, then by nights and weekends I was aspiring to be a full-time farmer. I know, what a swing in fields, but farming was my passion not sitting behind a desk.

As our relationship grew, Emily wanted more from me than just my hugs and kisses at night. She had transformed the idea of clocking in daily to run someone else's business, to the idea that she could be ready to start running her own family one day. This wasn't really something we spoke of a lot. No one we knew were having kids at the time. This made it difficult for her to see what they were going through, and if they loved being a mom or not.

Then take this as another sign, the country was now in turmoil. Corporate offices were letting employees work from home. The company that I worked for was all but non-existent now. The more time Emily and I spent together, the more she wanted to grow our family on the farm.

She could see the passion that I had when I would work the farm. She saw the love that I had for the animals and the land. This was making her want a family more than ever. The topic of having children would come up from time to time more often now. I was all for it as long as she was one hundred percent sure that's what she wanted.

My daughter from my previous partner, Clare, wasn't something that we had planned for when it happened. We weren't ready to be parents, but we had to be after we found out she was pregnant. This lack of planning threw a wrench into all the partying and fun things we were doing at the time. The pregnancy led to a lifestyle change that Clare and I were not ready for and didn't see coming so soon.

The pregnancy preplanning that Emily and I did was quite extensive. There were major shutdowns in the USA and you couldn't even get into a hospital if you wanted to. There were only certain providers that would take her insurance. Seeing as how my job was on the brink of extinction, I had limited insurance from work. I can't emphasize enough that you plan, plan and then make more plans, then you make backups for those plans.

Knowing that I never wanted to have a child in a hospital again. I made it pretty clear to Emily that we would need to have alternative places to go if necessary. We spent countless hours on the internet researching hospitals, birth centers and homebirth caretakers. We literally looked over every option and talked about each one.

The hospital that was local to us, was not the kind of place you would want to have a healthy child in. It was dirty, out of date and we knew the less than honest people that worked there. I was in their maternity ward after a friend had a baby several years ago. The experience wasn't that great. This hospital was not an option that I would choose.

Emily and I were both born in hospitals. I was born in a big city hospital. She was born in a small town one. We have nothing against a baby being born in a hospital. It's just our wishes to not have our child born in one. Especially after they lost Emily at birth and gave her back to the wrong mom! These are the variables that you can't control in a hospital.

After several interviews of local birth centers, we were less than pleased with the options that they had. To get into a nice one, we would have to drive an hour away. All to use the same room and tub that all the other women used to birth their children. While this isn't a big deal to most, Emily likes to be free to come and go as she feels necessary. She didn't want to make an appointment, to use a room, that may be unavailable on the day that the baby actually comes.

Having firsthand knowledge of a birth center, I was not keen on it either. My daughter was supposed to be born at a birth center. Clare and I had plans to have the baby on a certain week, when our midwife figured that the baby would be born. We already had our own sheets and blankets packed, along with the pillows and everything baby would need for an overnight stay. Clare even had a bottle of wine packed to help with her contractions.

We had the birthing center fully paid and ready to go. We didn't have insurance back then and they only would take payment for their services up front. Their fee was $5500 cash out of our pocket, with limited midwife assistance. I only say that it was limited because we had to pay for all tests, blood work, and certain exams in addition to their fee.

The best part of it was the resident midwife change a month before we were to deliver my little girl. Since it was a birth center, we ended up with a different midwife that was a smoker. It was pretty uncomfortable to be around a smoker when we were trying to have a healthy baby. The fact is that we were now in the care of a stranger that moved here from another state. She didn't seem as knowledgeable as the previous midwife we had. We both felt that we were receiving sub-par care now.

Being too late to find a new option to have the baby, we were stuck with the birthing center. We did not have the money to find another provider. I don't even think that another provider would take us a month before the due date.

In mine and Emily's own research, we had decided that the only place that we would have our child is at our home. Home is the place where our child would grow up, and could be proud to know they were born and raised in the same place. Home birth isn't an uncommon thing. Before there were hospitals on every corner, people actually had their children at home. I know this seems barbaric to some, but to us, it seemed to be the only option.

Keep in mind that we have done all this research before we ever made an attempt to conceive. I try to not make mistakes twice, and this homebirth option was becoming really important to Emily and I.

Chapter 3

Surprise I'm Pregnant

Can you ever be prepared for a surprise? With me, I can take a certain amount of surprise daily. Living on the farm, there is always a new surprise. Whether it is a new animal being born, or an injured one. You have to always be prepared for the unexpected.

The same holds true when you can hear the pitter patter of rabbit slippers headed toward you in the dark. The small whimpers that fill the room as she is headed your way! I could feel her getting closer from behind me. Her whimpers were growing stronger and stronger, as I turned around from the chair I was sitting in, while doing some work on the computer.

Her tears were rolling off her cheeks like a waterfall. All I could see was the glow she was radiating in the half dark room. Was there something wrong, I wondered? No, there was nothing wrong, she was glowing from the inside out. As that rabbit took its last step, I stood up just in time to catch her in my arms. "We're having a BABY" is all that she said, then I just held her. Emily's tears were soaking my shoulder as she squeezed me tighter. This might have been the happiest I've ever seen her. She was letting it all out now. "We are going to have a Baby" she expressed. I just held and kissed her on the top of her head. "Congratulations mom you've done it" I spoke in soft words into her ear.

This was the moment that I knew, this was what she really wanted. Emily would be a great mom to our child. This happened the night before Father's Day. Now I don't believe things happen by accident, I'm a firm believer that everything has a plan. If this was the plan that was made for me, then there was no better Father's Day gift in the world that anyone could ever give me.

You might ask yourself; "I wonder when they actually conceived the baby"? Good thing that in part of Emily's planning she made notes of just about everything you could imagine. From the food that we ate, to the amount of water we drank that day. She even jotted down the days that we made love. This made it easier to figure out about when the baby would be due. We had a pretty good idea when the baby was made. And the only way that we would truly know is from an early dating sonogram.

Seeing as we were so busy, there was only one of two places this took place. We both had a pretty good idea where it happened, but we would need to know for sure. *Do you really want to hear this part?* Ok, here goes. Emily had a business meeting close by my office that day. Since my company was on remote work only, the office was empty and I was the only one there. After her meeting she had come by to give me a kiss and hope that I was having a great day. Who would have guessed it turned into the day that I made my son.

I hope they don't fire me when they find out I made my baby at work. It's too late if they dislike my work ethics, my wife is more important to me than pushing paper for a living anyway.

With Clare, the reaction was slightly different. I found out that we were pregnant with my daughter 18 years ago. In 18 years, a man can change and so can the way he views situations. I was not the same man then as I am now. I was not ready to be a dad back then and Clare wasn't ready to be a mother either.

The way that I found out Clare was pregnant was different and more fitting to the situation at the time. It was Thanksgiving and we were having dinner at my folk's house. Clare was doing what some families do on a holiday. They drink and break bread to celebrate the holiday at hand.

Well Clare and I loved to drink. It was no surprise that she was washing down her turkey with a goblet of wine, that would be chased by a margarita or two just to keep her happy. I never liked liquor; I was more of a beer drinker.

While the party was cranking up pretty good, I've known Clare to never be sick no matter how much she had to drink. On this evening, it really was like a Thanksgiving to us. As much as we didn't plan for anything back then, Clare happened to have pregnancy tests in her overnight bag she called a purse. I didn't know at this point that she was pregnant or that she was taking a test. Why she even had them was beyond me at the time. I just figured that she was sick from eating too much or having one too many cocktails.

The bathroom door opened, and sure enough she was holding what appeared to be a pregnancy test in her hand. I wasn't seeing quite 20/20 vision at this point of the night, but I could tell from the way she was crying something was wrong. Clare had the look of fear on her face. It was not the type of look that I just experienced with my wife Emily.

Having a hard time even getting the words out, she blurted out, "Guess what?". I was thinking we were out of beer or something, but that was not the case. I was going to be a dad for the first time. It was in that moment that I instantly sobered up and a million things ran through my mind. We didn't have anything about our lives figured out yet, nor were we ready for the news that had just broken. One thing that we did have was a baby on the way.

It's kind of funny, that I can remember when I made my daughter. I remember the exact night, the exact place, and when it happened. I just can't remember the date. Somehow, we may forget things in life, but some things are meant to be memories that are kept forever.

I hope that you can remember important moments like this when they happen to you. It may be silly at the time, or even funny. As time passes by most people forget memories like that. If my daughter or son ever asked me where there were conceived. I could tell them the truth about it and feel confident that they would get the answer they were looking for.

I've asked my parents questions like that in the past. They barely remember the year I was born, let alone the place or day for that matter.

In part of the planning process that Emily and I have done, we accounted for things like this in the family journal. There will never be a question if our memories eventually fade.

Chapter 4

You're Pregnant, Now What?

Now is the best time to start getting your things in order! By order I don't mean getting your house tidied up! You are going to start doing your heavy research now. This is the stage that Emily really did her research. She started calling around to see availability on birth centers and midwifes that do homebirths.

There were tons of options when it came to hiring a professional to help us through the pregnancy. Could we have done it alone? I am pretty sure that most woman can, but there is always that cushion of knowing you have someone to answer your questions that makes the difference.

Emily has an OB that she uses for her woman care, but she has not been happy with the level of service they offered her currently and in the past. This provider was no longer an option that we were willing to rely on.

The insurance that we had would cover the child birth at an approved facility, less the large deductible. Emily called around to find the approved facilities that would accept us as clients. The idea of being stuck with a provider just because they accepted Emily's insurance was not an option in my book.

The thing is, we knew we would need someone that could offer the care that we were looking for and that they would be affordable. Similar to most families, we can't afford a lot of out-of-pocket bills and expenses in these rocky times. Heck, I could be only days away from not having a career anymore with the turmoil in the country.

Combining all of our research and experiences together, we had settled on the fact that we needed a midwife. She could help us have the birthing experience that we desired. This was not an easy task finding one either. Most of them were attached to the local birth centers and there were only a few that would do home births.

After several consultations we settled in on an appointment with a midwife that was within a 45-minute drive to our home. This seemed like a good idea as she would be able to get to us quickly, if needed.

Next came the interview process. Remember the midwife is not going to be your friend, she is your care provider. It didn't matter how young or old she was, what she looked like or how she dressed. All that we wanted was one that is well experienced in the field. One that could offer us their knowledge and the advice we needed to deliver our baby.

The interview went well and we hired her on the spot that day. She had availability to be our care provider and was willing to do mostly all of the appointments in our home. Now, there were some appointments that we had to go to her office for, like bloodwork and the first couple initial interviews.

While she could have taken our insurance, it wasn't guaranteed that it would be covered by the insurance company for a homebirth. I work hard for my money and so does Emily. The fact that we now had a new bill for the midwife that we just hired when we both had healthcare seemed kind of silly. I wasn't willing to put money ahead of my child's birth. It was way more important to me that we had the provider that we wanted, even though we would have to pay out of pocket. Luckily the midwife had a payment plan option that we used.

The process of finding a midwife now went a lot smoother than when I was looking for one 18 years ago with Clare. A midwife is a lot more accepted now than it was back then.

After the Thanksgiving surprise that Clare gave to me, we had to get our eggs in a row. We had to figure out how we were going to afford to have my daughter. I didn't have insurance back then and Clare was not working at the time. I made enough that we were able to afford to keep my daughter once she was born. The struggle to figure out how we would pay for the birth was a giant stress on our relationship.

I know it was a long time ago, but for some reason these details just seemed to etch themselves into me permanently. It's the kind of memories that I think you retain so that you won't be stuck in that situation again.

The interview process was pretty simple for this birth. There was only one birthing center and it was about an hour and twenty minutes away from our home. We had gone there to interview them and the place was great. They had several jacuzzi tubs and rooms with beds decorated in different colors depending on if you were having a boy or girl I'm guessing. The place presented very well.

They had two midwives on staff and several assistants to help. The place seemed perfect for having my daughter. I never even had a thought about a home birth at this time, that was out of the question. Clare was quite a bit older than me. She wasn't high risk or anything, she just wanted to have our daughter in a controlled environment where she had plenty of assistance. This was something that I was fine with.

We told the center that we would think about it over lunch and get back to them. The thing is, that we really didn't have the money to use their facility. Their package was $5500.00 and it was due in advance. This was quite the hill to climb in bare feet and we were seeming to just slide back down that hill.

I had made a call to several people I knew and they were not keen on lending me anything. My final call was to my sister and she agreed to lend me $5000.00 on a short-term loan. I was perfectly fine with that and agreed to repay her as soon as I could. I had a little bit of money in savings that would cover the rest of the blood work and other tests if needed.

There were also all of the upcoming bills that would be due now. We would now be putting baby stuff on my credit card. This can add a lot of stress to a man. Not to mention the stress that my family put on me for borrowing money to actually have the baby. FYI did I mention that the happiest moments in your life are always trying to be extinguished by the others around you! I hope that no one ever has to go through things like that.

Back to the birthing center we went with a check in hand. We needed to hire them so we would have a place to deliver the baby. This wasn't something we could handle on our own. Clare loved the main midwife; she was knowledgeable and very confident. I thought at that point we had made the right choice.

Both experiences had their positives and negatives. The older I get I tend to look for more of the positives in a situation than any of the negatives. The most positive thing to me is that we were having a baby, it is coming out one way or another. Might as well make your experience the best you can with what ever plan you decide to go with. That's exactly what I've done both times.

Chapter 5

In Office Bloodwork

The midwife that Emily and I chose, offered home visits. This was a major selling point for us. There were a few visits that were slated to be at her office though. Those were the initial consultation, along with the bloodwork that she suggested we have done. I am not going to get into the exact details of all the tests Emily had done, because honestly, she had only the basic ones completed and this wasn't an exciting event to me.

Options were available for hundreds of different things to look for in Emily's blood. We both agreed that we only wanted to know anything that would be pertinent to the safety of our child. This meant that we skipped all the fancy named tests, along with the boutique style tests that would tell us if our developing baby had genetic differences, that may show up later in life.

My opinion was that God sent us this child and I was willing to take whatever I was given. I already loved the baby and there was no looking back now. No test in the world would change my mind.

After this blood draw in office, we would just chat with the midwife about upcoming appointments and how the process would go throughout the pregnancy. With there not being a vaginal exam every appointment, this made for a more calming experience that put Emily at ease.

I really didn't mind going to her office, it wasn't like a birthing center, it was calm and peaceful. She had a little play area for parents to bring their other children when they had their visits. Along with a small book store that offered lots of books on birthing and health.

The exam room was cozy and friendly. It wasn't cold and industrial like a doctor's office would be. I can see why the midwife had a full schedule; she really was trying to create a better experience for families.

There was a discussion brought up about what events would take place that would make a homebirth not possible. This was very important to Emily and I as we knew what we wanted and we were going to get what we wanted.

The one condition that stuck with me the most was that she did not deliver breech babies. It was the way that she said it to me that left an impression. I know that she had a nice cozy office and that she seemed to be very well experienced, but honestly, she had no finesse.

This came out like this: "I do not deliver breech babies, if your baby is breech you will be transferred to the hospital". Some way to win over a new client. I would have thought that she could have explained how the babies will turn on their own if they are breech towards the end of pregnancy. Besides, it was too early to even be talking of this, but I understand that she was just making us aware.

After my experiences and the fact that you're still reading this book, I will say that your provider will most likely, at some point in time, try to scare you in some way. Don't take it personally, they are just doing their job. Remember, they are not your friend; they are just your provider.

This was the last visit we would have at her office for a while. The next visit would be at home. This made it easier for me to take the day off of work and stay home to be the support partner that Emily needed.

Chapter 6

Baby's First Sonogram Week 9

This was an option that we were made aware of by the midwife.

There are rules attached when you hire a care provider. With the midwives in our state, there are windows of time when they can deliver a baby in their care. These rules apply to before the agreed upon due date and after the due date.

I can't stress this fact enough! You need to know pretty precisely when your baby will be due.

Emily and I were not 100 percent sure on the actual conception date. We had two possible dates that we could have made him on the calendar. We wanted to be absolutely sure which one it was. Calculating from her last period, we knew that it could have been one of only two dates, that we conceived our little man. What couldn't be taken into account was that she never had a regular period with a date pattern that was reliable. This made it almost impossible to get the exact conception date.

This being the case, we could end up not having a midwife there to help us with the birth if we had our son to early or too late. This was something that haunted me from Clare's pregnancy and was a big concern to me.

The midwife suggested that we have a dating sonogram to determine how far along Emily was. Then the delivery window could be set in stone. From past experience, there is no leeway in their dating process. Once the midwife picks your due date, they set the expiration date for their services.

Time was of the essence to get the dating sonogram scheduled. The midwife had a sonographer that she recommended. The dating scan will tell you when the baby was conceived pretty precisely. There is a small window of time that you have to complete this dating sonogram and the deadline was fast approaching.

We interviewed the sonographer and she was pretty great. She was even willing to do an in-home visit. Her results would be uploaded to our midwife so that the proper delivery date could be established.

This experience was fantastic, no traveling to an office far away. Just make the appointment and the lady brought all of the equipment right into our home. This was a great weight off of our shoulders as we still had to be at work and didn't have all day to travel for a scan.

Emily and I decided that we didn't want to overdo the number of sonograms that we would expose our little baby to. This one just happened to be necessary. It would secure the date that our baby would be born, within the time frame that we were now allotted.

With Clare, there was a sonogram, but 18 years ago they just went off your last period and set a date in stone. This proved to be a failure as far as I was concerned. Clare didn't even know when her last period was, so her and the midwife just picked a date and used that. Now this was not science as far as I was concerned. I wasn't really keen on the way they did this and it would prove to be disastrous later on in the pregnancy.

My experience with Clare and the birthing center already seemed like a pretty invasive event. Every time we would go to her appointments, they would do a vaginal exam and want to hear the baby's heartbeat. Now this may not seem too invasive to some, but I'm sure that my baby girl, growing inside of Clare, wasn't keen on having the sound wave bouncing off of her every visit.

I feel that the experience I've had with Emily has been a world of change from the one with Clare. I owe this to our research, planning and knowing what Emily and I actually want as a family.

Chapter 7

I Freaking Quit! 11 Weeks In

There is no better feeling than to know that you have made your own choices. Now, sticking by them takes team work with your other half. You have to stick by the plans you made and don't let others break you down with their idea that you can't do something. You really can do anything that you put your mind to. Emily did.

Just a short time ago we received the happiest news of our lives. Emily was pregnant! We were going to be parents together. This news trumped all of the other silly things that happened in our day to day lives. The thought of her carrying my baby was so exciting to me. She just cried for hours over it. This was the happiest I've seen her in some time! I would never let anyone take that happiness from her.

Remember that awesome job Emily loved at the Fortune 500 company? Well, as amazing as she was at it and she really did put her all into it. They couldn't compete with the new job that she was about to take. They had no idea that she took this new job a little more seriously than theirs.

After the tears subsided, from the initial shock of finding out we were going to be parents, something had changed inside of Emily. I could see it on her face and I could feel it in her heart. She was no longer going to be that career woman that I met just a few years ago. She had this new career that was paving the way for her to declare her independence.

The firm that she worked for would no longer be able to put their unneeded stress on her as they no longer owned her. This baby now owned her and she knew it! This is what Emily wanted deep down inside of her soul. Corporate America couldn't have her valuable time anymore.

I knew what I wanted for my family and it was that we be together and work for a future as a family. Spend as much time together as we could in the early parts of my child's life. Give the opportunity for a stress-free home that my child could prosper in.

31

This wasn't going to work with the untold stresses that were put on Emily's plate every day by the corporate world. They didn't know she was pregnant, she never told them. This was our family it was none of their business.

The lack of respect that the corporate overlords offered Emily was starting to put untold stress on her. I could see it daily as I would come home from work. I didn't let stress get to me like she did. I just let stress roll off my shoulders and well, she seemed to hold it in. The stress couldn't be healthy for our child that was being made in her womb.

We didn't have a plan on how to replace her corporate income or the health insurance that she carried through them. But we did have a plan to be happy and stress free. That was our plan.

The discussions we had were of bringing down her stress level and not letting any of the anger from work pass to our growing baby. This could only be accomplished by not being their slave anymore.

It was a corporate meeting earlier in the week that would set the ball into motion for the end of Emily's corporate relationship. They didn't know anything about Emily. Just that she was a name on their corporate roster and she had a certain quota to meet. Well, she always met her quota, and everyone loved her in her position.

Those who are too good at their jobs will never advance in the corporate world. They will leave you in that position until you retire if they can. They had big plans to double Emily's work load with no fair compensation to match the work. We had discussed the events that took place at the meeting, and I was less than pleased with what their strategies were.

It was this next move that made Emily a free woman and she has never been the same woman since. Come Friday, she had decided that she would not do twice the work for the same pay. Inflation was killing us already and the price of everything was going through the roof. Her firm was raising their rates, but not offering the staff any extra for the consolidations and extra work they piled on their staff.

Never planning that this event would take place, we really were not prepared for it. This would change the way we lived. Change our lifestyle and change our ability to have a little extra in our pockets.

None of that mattered to me. The only thing that mattered was the health of my child and Emily. The amount of rollover sick time, the vacation time she had banked up and the 12 weeks paid maternity leave didn't even sway her to keep the position at the firm.

It was Friday the 13th, how ironic is that? Emily woke up and said this is the day. I've had enough of their stress and just can't do it anymore. We talked about her options one last time and the only thing that mattered to us was the baby, nothing else.

Taking no time at all, Emily drafted her resignation letter and sent it off to her boss and the HR department. Just a few minutes later, I heard her phone ring. The decision was now final, Emily had made the decision to choose her family over her career. Her now previous boss was on the phone throwing around deals to save Emily's position at the firm. This was an oversight on their part! They should have thought about the worth of their employee before bringing them to the point of leaving with no notice.

Emily is not the type of woman to ever quit anything, she is the strongest woman I know. Her choice to end the relations she had with the stress machine, was one that I will never hold against her. It was a decision that I am very proud of her for making!

Chapter 8

First At Home Visit 15 Weeks

Being the first at home appointment, we didn't know what to expect. We were about to find out though. There was no glitz and glamour. The midwife shows up, you greet her, show her into the living room and the talking begins. You are doing the talking while she seems to be writing your whole life story into a word document on her laptop computer.

At first, I was under the impression that we hired the midwife to deliver our baby, but at this point it would seem that she was in the business of charting on her laptop. To make a file on Emily, I would assume.

First thing was first. The standard vital signs were taken. Blood pressure and heart rate would be charted, along with asking just a few questions.

Then the midwife pulled out this doppler thing that looked like a mini sonogram tool. She placed it on Emily's belly and sure enough there was a heartbeat. Boy was it pumping, our baby had a great heartbeat. Knowing that we didn't want our baby to be tested for anything that wasn't vital or required by law, we also didn't want these tools used unless they were necessary.

This would be the only visit that we would allow her to use the doppler to hear the heartbeat. There is another option that we knew of that is called a fetoscope. This is a stethoscope looking thing that makes it slightly more difficult to find the heartbeat, but it's in no way invasive and offers no harm to the baby. This was something that was on our research list that wasn't debatable. This method would be the new standard for us.

The midwife then went over Emily's bloodwork results from the previous office visit. There were no comments on any of the results, everything was in range. There were no concerns to be spoken of. Emily was in great shape and in great health going into the pregnancy. She didn't smoke or drink. She even exercised from time to time. She was the perfect person to have an at home birth.

Next came the viewing of the results of the dating sonogram. This would change the due date by two weeks in that fancy system the midwife used for charting and tracking. Turns out, we went to our first consultation thinking that the pregnancy was two weeks further along than it actually was. Now that the results were medically proven we had to adjust the due date backwards by 2 weeks.

The midwife would only change the due date because we had this early scan that proved how far along the baby actually was. If we did not do the scan we might have timed out of her care before the baby could have delivered. This takes us back to that rule of 2 weeks before the due date and two weeks after the due date that is absolutely ridiculous.

The discussion also came up that the midwife would now need to drop the insurance provider on record, as Emily was no longer employed. This meant that we would have no chance of recovering any reimbursement toward the birthing or lab work costs from the insurance company.

The rest of the home visit was just chatting about our next appointment and what to expect until that appointment comes. This early in the pregnancy there really wasn't anything to expect. It was noted that any correspondence that we would do with the midwife should be through the online portal. We were given access to the portal for adding notes to Emily's chart.

The way that we took that was to not text or call the midwife with any questions or concerns. Rather we should address them to the file so that they could be addressed formally. The midwife was pretty emphatic that she could offer better service if we contacted her through this portal not over text or phone.

We never bothered the midwife with any questions or concerns up to this point that would need to be logged into the online portal. Instead, we just made a list of questions to ask when she was in person. Honestly, the home visits were not exciting in any way. There was never anything brought up at this point that we really didn't know. All of our research up until now covered all the questions that we had. The home visits just weren't very exciting.

The main thing that I did notice throughout the visits was that our midwife would change the schedule on us quite a bit. This could pose a problem for anyone that has to take off work to be home. I had to change my schedule quite a bit to meet the new schedule as it was changed on very short notice.

Don't get freaked out if your provider is tired when they arrive at your home, or if they don't seem to be taking in everything that you're talking about. This happened several times to us. Fact is that the providers deliver babies at all hours of the day and night. If your appointment happens to be after one of their all-nighter's, you may be slightly aggravated with the level of professionalism you receive. This early on there wasn't really anything that we needed to discuss of importance.

Chapter 9

Anatomy Scan Week 19

Now was the time that we started to take an interest in keeping Emily's skin moisturized. This was something that we pre-planned to do anyway. Listening to podcasts and reading books we knew that if we prevented her skin from stretching it may not tear.

Trying several lotions, nothing really seemed to keep her moisturized very well, as her little baby bump started to grow. This led us in many directions to make sure that she didn't get stretch marks on her belly or breasts.

The last thing we tried was organic coconut oil. This stuff was amazing it soaked in fairly quickly. When her skin had enough it could just be wiped off with a cotton towel. This process was a nightly event that rarely was forgotten. Her hormones were raging and I think that she just wanted an excuse for me to touch her.

I can't stress enough to not skip the lotion process! During Emily's last three days of pregnancy, she did start to get small stretch marks. She has seven tiny marks now that do not look bad at all. If we didn't moisturize, I feel that she would have had a whole lot more of them.

Next on the schedule was the anatomy scan. This was one of the most exciting parts of the pregnancy so far. We were now 19 weeks into this pregnancy and we had something to really look forward to.

Up until now we had only heard the heartbeat to reassure us that the baby was safe and growing. What a better way to encourage us as parents than to give a sneak peek into our child's life inside the womb. This is just the encouragement we needed to keep eating healthy and exercising. This will be the closest view into what our baby looks like and is developing into.

The scheduling process for the anatomy scan was very easy. The sonographer would just text message back and forth to set up the appointment and the date was set.

Now if you're planning on having an audience to see this you may want to warn them that not everyone in the baby business can be on time all the time. She was running an hour late due to traffic, but was right on top of updating us as she was slowly headed our way. Now we didn't have anyone coming over to see the anatomy scan. We felt this was the first time we were getting to really see the baby and we wanted that moment to be special to us.

As promised, she did finally show up and I helped lug all of her equipment into the house. It was setup in the living room now and I had to run a cord from our television to her computer to act as a monitor. This was pretty great; we were going to be able to see the baby on our own television. How great of an experience this was becoming!

Emily laid down on the couch and pulled up her shirt just above her baby bump. I lowered the lights and closed all the blinds. This was like movie night and my new child was going to be the star. A few squirts from her clear liquid bottle and the lady started working her magic wand. I began to see what resembled body parts on the tv as Emily squeezed my hand harder.

This was it! We were just moments away from finding out if I made a boy or a girl. I was pretty excited. Emily had what looked to be moisture accumulating around her eyes, she was about to cry.

The excitement started to build as the lady looked over the spine first. She was pounding keys on her keyboard and marking measurements like she was drawing a map. She narrated as to what she was measuring and why. The most fulfilling part was hearing her play by play as the event carried on.

Not knowing what the results might turn out to be, I can say that there was a small amount of anxiousness that was brewing inside of me. Trying to watch the tv screen and Emily's face at the same time seemed daunting and pretty hard to do. Then throw in that I was trying to shoot pictures of the tv with my phone at the same time. This was exciting and a full-time job all wrapped into one.

The sonographer sure knew what she was doing. She would talk to the baby as she moved that wand around and the baby seemed to listen. There was one view where she was checking the condition of the cord and the baby literally wrapped its hands around the freaking cord. I can't make this stuff up; it really was happening right in front of my eyes.

Then she really started to get into the vital organs, recording them on her laptop. She was like a robot at this point. She was banging keys on the keyboard, explaining what we were seeing and talking to the baby all at the same time. This lady really knew her business.

Next came the money shot. That's right the part we had waited all too long to know. As she inched down the baby's belly, there it was, The Family Jewels! I've never seen Emily cry so hard from sheer happiness. She was bawling her eyes out and her little tummy was shaking. I could just feel the love in the air as the lady said "I hope you ordered a BOY". I nodded my head towards her and thanked her for the great news.

We wanted a boy all along. That is what we prayed for before we even made him and our prayers were now answered.

There was still a lot of scanning the lady had to do. We were only about half way into the 45-minute session when we received the great news. The more the sonographer talked to him, the more he did what she wanted him to do. He seemed to be listening to her when she needed him to turn to his other side so she could view him better.

Somehow, I believe that he could hear us as we spoke to him. Perhaps he just wanted her to turn the machine off so he could get some rest. He seemed to be hurrying the process along for her. No matter what the case may be, I just found out that we are having a Boy and that made me very happy.

As the session was ending, he was in the breech position. That meant that he was feet down if he wanted to come out. This was noted on the file. We have read that a baby can turn on their own when they are ready. This wasn't a concern to us at all. He was only 19 weeks into his journey, a lot could change in the next 20 weeks.

Chapter 10

More Office And Home Visits

The fun was all over now! Not really, the fun was just beginning. We were going to have a baby soon and that is all that we cared about.

The next visit from the midwife was at our home. It consisted of her measuring Emily's stomach to see how many inches our baby boy was now and completing the standard checks. Emily stood on our scale and gave her weight. Next came her blood pressure and pulse check. Everything was normal as usual nothing to really talk about.

Preparing yourself for an hour-long visit can be slightly daunting when there is nothing to talk about. I tried to sit in on every visit that I could to support Emily. Apparently, I can be slightly intimidating with my rough voice and strong tone, so I tried to keep my mouth shut as much as I could.

We were not onboard to have the doppler used to check the baby's heart rate. This seemed like a lot to constantly hit him with waves that he didn't need. I will say that the midwife always brought her fetoscope and had to do it the old-fashioned way. The baby's heart was always strong and there were really no concerns that Emily or I had this far in the pregnancy.

The midwife would look through her laptop and go over the same things every visit. She would just ask general questions like, how are you feeling and have you been drinking enough fluids. Well, in fact Emily was drinking 7-8 bottles of water at the minimum each day. That was a lot for her to get down, especially after you take into account that she was also drinking 32 ounces of fruit smoothie with that.

The only concern that was raised by the midwife was that Emily didn't urinate while she was here for the hour appointment. She didn't know the size of Emily's bladder either. Emily can hold a lot of fluids in her body and that seems to help keep her hydrated.

The midwife did show us a few stretching techniques that we could do around the house to stretch Emily out and get her muscles ready for the baby.

I know that the midwife we hired was trying to do what she learned in school and from her own experience. Emily on the other hand wasn't like a lot of women, she was built different than most. Well, you won't learn that in an hour-long session once a month, or from the chart that the midwife was keeping on her laptop.

There really wasn't a lot of questions raised about Emily's day to day life or if she was able to drink a lot of fluids before she became pregnant. That's why I mentioned the part about the midwife or care provider just being there to be of service to you. They are not your friend. Your friends will know more about your life than anyone.

The next visit was another blood draw at the midwife's office. This consisted of the same questionnaire as the last visit, along with a blood draw to be sure that there were no deficiencies in Emily. Emily and the midwife just chatted as if it was a get to know you session so they could get more acquainted with each other.

When I used to go to the office visits at the birth center with Clare, they were much more involved with her. Clare took it upon herself to befriend everyone she met, so there was a lot more conversation that went on there. Also, like I said previously, Clare had a vaginal exam almost every visit.

Vaginal exams every visit was something that Emily and I didn't want unless necessary. Turns out that it's ok to just say no. Just because you are offered something does not mean that you have to do it.

Emily and I knew what we wanted. We wanted a baby born as naturally as possible in our home. We did not want all the extras that were offered like the vitamin shots, ointments and whatever herbs and pills were available. We declined everything that wasn't mandatory by our state law, or required to stay in the care of the midwife.

Emily and I worked really hard to do our research on all the prenatal pills, vitamins and minerals that the baby would need. This proved that we were on the right track. The lab then sent the results of the blood work to the online chart, that we had to look at ourselves. (Go figure) Iron levels were spot on and her vitamin D was far from being deficient. The midwife never called about it so we figured there was nothing wrong. Surely there were no problems with Emily's blood.

Going into the at home birth we knew that we would need a midwife that was not very thorough. That's why we hired who we did. She was a very nice woman, seemed to take her practice seriously, but I could tell just how spread thin she was. The good news was that she was only spread thin in the months leading up to our due date. February was the month that our boy was due and she had minimal clients booked for that month.

Emily and I knew that if she got the bulk of her other births done before we were due, we would get better service from her when we needed her. That's exactly how it seemed to play out.

There were a few trying times that I wanted to fire her. I questioned why we even needed a midwife to begin with. She was pretty abrupt on things. Well, it's kind of hard to throw stuff at Emily when she is emotional, and it's even harder to throw stuff at me when I'm on edge.

After a quick glance over the 19-week sonogram results it was clear that the baby was breech. So, the midwife brought that up at a couple visits. She was emphatic that she did not deliver breech babies. So, when our meeting was over, I would tell Emily how her lack of compassion toward things was really making want to fire her.

This was a scenario that happened 4 times throughout the whole process with the midwife. Now, don't let me scare you about the process. Babies turn on their own when they're ready, according to all the research we have done. You can even spin them if needed. Now, she did offer the advice on how to spin the baby after stating that she does not deliver breech babies. So that saved our relationship on that visit.

Well, I guess that there must have been some kind of miss communication in the fact that, Emily and I were going to deliver this baby! She was just going to be there to chart the event and make sure that the baby wasn't in distress in any way. To me it didn't really matter what position the baby was in. Emily and I were not depending on anyone, but ourselves, to keep our baby safe through the birthing process.

Our baby boy turned on his own when he was good and ready like most do. Your care provider can try to intimidate you along the way. Just remember you always have the ultimate say in the way you choose to birth your child. Emily and I did.

The secret that I learned from home birth is, the mom delivers the baby on her own. The midwife, her assistant and anyone else that is there, including the dad, does not deliver the baby. Mom does all the work; we are all just there as witnesses to watch the event. It is our job to cheer on mom and make her as happy and comfortable as possible throughout this journey of child birth.

Chapter 11

Meeting The Assistant

Hello February!

The final month is here and wouldn't you know that the baby will be here soon. We had what would have been one of our last weekly visits scheduled and the midwife happen to fall ill. Now, I will say that I was very grateful that she contacted us and offered another option for the appointment that was scheduled.

The last thing we needed was for Emily to be around anyone that was sick. The whole pregnancy from the time she left her position at the fortune 500 company until now, we had limited contact with anyone that was even remotely ill in any way.

This pregnancy meant the world to Emily and I. There were no social events or places we needed to be that were more comfortable to us then home.

The midwife was able to send her assistant for a meet and greet and a get to know her session. This was a great idea, in fact, we were glad that we had the opportunity to meet with her before the actual birth.

Emily had a great connection with the assistant. She showed her around our home to get her familiar with what she would be working with on birthing day.

They went room to room and made her familiar with where we would be delivering the baby. Even showed her the bath tub that we would be using to birth our child together. They also went over the birthing kit. This was required that we buy on our own. It was not something that the midwife supplied.

The vibe that this woman, the assistant Laura, put off was friendly and enthusiastic. I wanted her to come to all the appointments from now on with the midwife. Her upbeat tone and confidence made Emily grateful that she hired the midwife to begin with.

From the moment Emily saw her, Laura was glowing from the inside out. I could see Emily feeding off of her energy. She made Emily so at ease. I was really grateful that she had come that day.

For the first time in the pregnancy Laura was the first one that asked Emily what her wishes were in the birth. Did she have a certain way that she pictured things going?

Was there a scenario that Emily would like to be the perfect scenario?

This being the first time that she was asked this; she was falling in love with the idea of Laura coaching her through the labor. Laura understood Emily. She was only feeding her good energy and was just there to help. It was an all-new feeling that Emily needed to open up her mind to the way that she would carry out the birth.

Emily explained that she wanted her and I to work through everything together until the baby would come out into her arms. Emily was only wanting the midwife to step in if there was a major issue that we both missed. The vibe that Laura put off that day stuck with Emily. After Laura touched Emily's belly, she said the baby is ready at any time now.

Is there an actual vibe that people put off to make you happy or sad? Yes, there is. In our case the flood gates were opened in Laura's presence. Emily was so happy to be having our son that she just couldn't wait for him to come out now.

I don't know if Laura was a good luck charm or just an angel, that was sent to raise Emily's spirits in the delivery of our baby son. Either way I'm grateful she was here.

The entire visit was peaceful, there was no bad energy in our home. Emily was finally at peace with the fact that we had made the right choice, with who we hired to help with our at home delivery.

At the end of our home visit, Laura used the fetoscope to listen to baby's heart. As she measured Emily's belly for the last time, it was like her energy was passing into Emily. That energy would give her that final round of confidence she would need to keep going in this last month of pregnancy.

I can't stress enough that you need to have positive people around you when you're pregnant. Anyone that isn't positive needs to hit the road. Emily and I would not let anyone bring us down in this pregnancy, even though several tried. We only associated with happy people and wanted all the good energy from their happiness to transfer into the baby.

Laura showed Emily how to make ice packs and get them pre-frozen for when she was in labor. She also had a few suggestions on how labor was going to be.

Now, I know that we hired a midwife, but with her came the assistant. The assistant would help at birth with all the silly stuff that we couldn't handle while the baby was on its way. Her tasks even included the final clean up after baby came. This would allow us to spend as much time bonding with the baby as possible uninterrupted.

With Clare, when my daughter was born in the hospital, we didn't have any of these clean up tasks that would need to be completed. At the birthing center, they had assistants that were going to offer the same services to us. Unfortunately, we never had the opportunity to use their services after they transferred us to the hospital from the birthing center.

Chapter 12

Waterfalls From Heaven

We had a lot going on in our life for the past several months. It seemed like everyone wanted to throw their drama at us. There seemed to never be a break and we were busier than we had ever been. When you get to the point that you think you're going to have a moment to breathe, someone or something throws more projects at you. This just seems to be the normal for us anymore.

I had it set in my mind that the baby would be born in early March, after all the work that piled onto us would be throttled back. Emily's sister was starting her divorce and she had a young child herself. That opened the door to lots of drama and hard work to help her move and get re-situated with her life.

Just because we were excited to welcome our baby boy into the world and our life was going great; doesn't mean that everyone else's is. Emily and I are not selfish in any way. We never leave someone to be on their own when they need us. We are always there for them.

Our parents are getting older and that makes an added workload trying to help them out when we can. There are always projects that get thrown my way what seems to be weekly, if not daily. Perhaps it's our parents' way of spending more time with me and Emily?

Then there are the random friends and family that constantly have stuff they need help with. It would seem that when you try to make more time for yourself, someone finds a way to use it for you. We usually don't mind taking on their burdens, except for the fact that, Emily is now ready to birth our child any day. She can't handle the heavy lifting and endurance work anymore.

Working late on Friday night at the home computer; I was dosing off and Emily shooed me off to bed. Up I would go half asleep, to brush my teeth and get tucked in for the night. Already suffering from sleep deprivation, I was struggling to keep my eyes open. Emily was in the shower after she had just shut down the house for the evening.

Normally, she will lay next to me and kiss me goodnight before I pass out. That didn't happen on this Friday night, I think I was snoring with my eyes still open. I couldn't have been asleep for more than about ten minutes or so before my whole life changed.

The best way I can explain what happened next is when you're dead asleep and a fire alarm goes off. You jump up from a dead sleep to see what the heck is going on and you're in shock.

Well, that was my fate at 12:30AM Saturday morning. With the long week finally behind me, I was going to get some sleep. Getting some sleep meant I wouldn't have to be up until 3:00AM to let our dogs out to pee. I had no sooner fallen asleep, when I heard the sound that I don't ever want to hear again. It was a sound of fear, pain and excitement all in one. It was like I was dreaming and I didn't believe what I was hearing.

Up I went as fast as I could. "What's wrong?" I yelled. Emily cried, "come here please, come here now". As I made my way into the bathroom, she was sitting on the toilet pointing down. My boxer brief underwear that she always wore to bed were soaking wet. I said "what happened? did you pee yourself?", While I was gazing at Emily with one eye pried open in that well-lit bathroom.

She said my eyes were bloodshot and I looked like a zombie. Well, wake an exhausted man up and that's what you get!

"I think my water just broke", she said in her serious voice. I looked at her and could tell, just by the look on her face, the tears she had on her cheeks were happy ones.

There was no sadness to be had. She said, "the baby is coming, we are going to finally meet our son". I'm thinking that maybe that good vibe was still inside of Emily from when Laura visited and touched her belly. You couldn't ever take away the happiness that I saw on her face that early Saturday morning.

Emily, in her tears of happiness, was in shock to what just happened. She was prepared for a different feeling when her water broke. Reading up on the subject previously, she was expecting to hear a pop or something dramatic happen. Like she would be at the grocery store and it would happen there. Not at home before bed.

Not her luck for any such event like that to happen. She was just brushing her teeth when her water broke. Just standing there looking in the mirror brushing away when the warm sensation filled my dark blue boxer briefs. This happened just a moment before I heard the scream, yes, that scream.

Staring at her, as she sat on the toilet and more fluid was coming out, I asked "did you just pee yourself?". She was emphatic that her water broke. I wasn't so sure. I figured maybe the baby was pushing on something and she just peed herself. I was asked to smell it and feel it to see if it was pee. Like a good husband, I went for it. It didn't have a smell and it had what looked to be a small amount of a membrane in it.

OH BOY, it was getting pretty real now. I grabbed my phone and looked up what the amniotic fluid is supposed to look and smell like. The search said that if it was smelly, we have a problem. If it was not smelly, we were probably in a better situation. That was relieving for me to know that it was clear, with no odor and looked like pee.

I was telling Emily to just come to bed and we will see what happens in the morning. She wouldn't go for that though. I really was having trouble keeping my bloodshot eyes open.

When I bought the midwife required supplies for our birthing kit, I made sure to buy a lot of extra stuff. It was on the list that we have *qty:1 Amino swab*. Well, this tricky little cotton swab looking thing can tell you whether your water has broken or not. They had a 10 pack and that's what I got.

Heading off to the spare bedroom to get these swabs out of the birthing kit, my mind was full of thoughts. I was replaying in my mind how if this thing is positive, it will be a very long weekend. If it is not positive, then I will get to finally sleep. I grabbed them out of the plastic tote and headed back to the bathroom where Emily was still crying.

Opening the first one I read the directions. It said to insert this thing inside of her and rub around. Well, no offense, but I don't know where the heck these things were made. I wasn't about to put it inside of anything. I dabbed the swab on the overly soaked boxer briefs and almost instantly it was positive. Her water had broken.

Now I'm more of a best out of three kind of guy. I don't like to rely on one test for anything. I ran to the kitchen and got a clear glass bowl. I had Emily hold it under her as more fluid leaked from her. This was as fresh as it was going to get and it was not urine.

In the interim, while waiting on Emily to leak more fluid, I saw a small amount of fluid that she had leaked on the bathroom floor. I took another swab out of the plastic packaging and rolled it through the fluid. It was almost instant and the swab turned dark color. I compared it to the chart and sure enough, her water was broken.

Now, I'm not great at following instructions, but there was still no way I was going to put these things inside of her! I do know that when you test something a couple times and they all say the same thing, it's a pretty good chance that they're not wrong.

With Clare and my daughter this was not the case at all. I don't have a great story about how the water broke, or how there was a whole event attached to it. Her water was broken by a random hospital staff member. What I can tell you is that it was pretty invasive.

They used a long skinny red tool that had a hook at the end of it to break Clare's water. She was laying on her back in the hospital bed and had her feet up flat on the bed. The nurse lady inserted this thing inside of Clare and the lady pulled really hard and nothing happened. So, she had to do it several times until the actual water broke. It was an event that I will not forget as it didn't look very safe. I was concerned they would hurt my daughter.

Then within a few minutes they took a tool with a wire attached to it and screwed it into my daughter's head. Now this was freaking me out! My daughter was now attached to a monitor through a wire that was screwed into her head. I was not happy about this at all.

At this point of the night, we were pretty sure that Emily's water has broken. Emily's mother was only in labor with her for two hours before she was born. This led me to believe that this baby could come at any moment. Emily had to remind me that she hadn't even had a contraction yet. This process was going to take more than two hours for sure.

Emily headed in to lay on the bed as more water was leaking from her. She laid down for a moment and I put my ear to her belly. Moving my ear around, it was only on her left side that I could hear the baby's heartbeat. It was fast and strong. I knew that he was ok and still safe inside of his mom.

This was the point that the adrenaline started to fuel me. There was so much to do if this baby was coming and I was far from ready. I grabbed a cup from the cabinet and made myself a coffee with an extra splash of sugar. I needed a rush of energy to get my chores done.

Creating a list inside of my head, I was 6 hours away from finishing the chores that I just willed to myself. It was now 12:45AM on Saturday morning and the countdown had just begun.

Emily was on the computer trying to figure out why she was not having contractions, but her water had broken.

Turns out that this happens to only six percent of moms and there was no good explanation why.

The baby crib was in the wrong room and would need to be moved. Emily was busy researching and couldn't help me. Plus, she couldn't lift anything she was about to be in labor. Grabbing a few towels, I put them under the legs of the crib and drug this thing through the house, scratching the floor along my path. I didn't care that I was being haphazard. I wanted to get ready for our baby.

The dishes were piled high in the sink and the laundry was far from being done. The toilets needed to be cleaned and the sinks sanitized. Both of the beds would need to have double sheets installed with liners. I had a long night ahead of me.

Starting in the kitchen, I ran through the dishes and had them piled up to dry. It sure would have been nice to just throw them in the dishwasher, but ours was out of service.

Off to clean the toilets I went; I saw a lot of birth stories where woman would deliver their child on the toilet. There was no way I would have my baby poking his head around in a dirty crapper. Not wanting to use chemicals or bleach around Emily or the baby, I grabbed the oxy stuff from the laundry room and went to town polishing the porcelain. I think it's probably the cleanest the toilets have ever been.

I told Emily that we need to buy more of this stuff it worked so well.

Going from bedroom to bedroom, I added an extra layer of mattress protectors and another set of sheets to each bed. Just in case we would need to do a fast change.

Next, I started banging out the laundry. I knew that we would need tons of towels and support linens to get through this ordeal. While I was playing Mr. housewife, Emily was in and out of the shower from the fluid leaking down her leg. She was doing more research to find out when she would go into labor, when to call the midwife and so on. She was now leaking fluid on the computer chair as well.

Thing is, there was never a discussion with the midwife on when to call her or ask for help. Being 2:30 in the morning now, we were not about to wake anyone up if we didn't know that we needed them.

Laura had given Emily a small set of contraction standards that she used to determine when to call the midwife. Emily had only just started to feel a small flutter in her lower stomach that felt less than a period cramp.

At this point I took over control of the computer. The last load of laundry was in the washer. I felt that I had succeeded in getting the house in order for the baby's arrival. I was searching any and everything I could to find out if we could go back to bed. That cup of coffee was wearing off and I was about done.

I added a few layers of towels on Emily's side of the bed. It was now just after 3:00AM and I needed to close my bloodshot eyes and take a nap. My body was on high alert and I was sleeping with one eye open to keep watch over Emily and my baby. The restlessness set in. Every time Emily would move or grunt, I would awake to check on her. Then the dogs would bark and I would have to let them outside.

The next three hours we were able to sleep. That small amount of rest would have to take us until our child was born.

Chapter 13

That Saturday Morning

The lack of sleep was one thing, but waking up to Emily still not in labor was pretty trying on my conscious. One would think that there is something wrong. I leaned into her belly with my ear again, listening to hear if my son still had a heartbeat. Sure enough, it was as strong as ever. His heart was echoing off of my ear drum. I was tapping my fingers on Emily's arm so that she could feel how fast his heart was beating.

In the birthing kit that we put together; I purchased a stethoscope to have just in case. While I tried over and over to hear his little heartbeat; the only thing that I could hear was the sound of a washing machine that about matched the heart rate of Emily. Upon further research on the computer, turns out that was also good to hear. That unmistakable sound was fluid passing through the umbilical cord from the placenta into my baby.

It's pretty satisfying to be able to hear what's going on inside of Emily. Especially to not have it done with a fancy medical machine. I was sure now that my baby boy was safe and he would come when he was good and ready. Emily and I were ready for him to come, but he sure wasn't.

Her contractions felt no different than light period cramps. She was commenting how easy this was and how she could do this all day long. Well, watch what you wish for you just might get it.

Our morning seemed to fly by and before I knew it, lunch would have to be made. I decided that I better make plenty of extra, so that we had it on hand if this process drug on for a while.

Emily was bouncing on her birthing ball and walking laps around the house; while I was prepping for lunch. Soup and mashed sweet potatoes were on the menu. They would be easy to eat and provide energy. I even made Emily a red raspberry leaf tea to help her move things along.

I peeled the potatoes first and set them at a slow rolling boil. While they were working, I started to cut up celery, onion, carrots, green beans and parsley. This was my usual vegetable soup recipe. I also added in pasta noodles for the carbs Emily would need to push through the labor. The potatoes were done now, I drained the water off then added butter and brown sugar to them. Mashing away I had a million things running through my head about how this would all work out.

Emily and I wanted our son born during the day, not at night. This was just a preference that we had, but it wasn't necessary. We were still in labor at this point, just not heavy labor yet.

I was folding laundry and finishing the dishes that I had made from lunch. Emily was trying to bounce on her ball and walk as much as she could. I had soothing music playing throughout the house to help keep her calm and ease the contractions that were growing stronger.

At this point no one knew that Emily was in labor. We had decided that telling anyone would take away the peacefulness that we had in our home. Since the midwife never told us when to let her know Emily was in labor, we figured why add any stress onto us. We decided we would just wait and call her if we needed her.

The only thing that we needed at this point was to work on Emily being comfortable and for her to focus on delivering the baby.

I gave her some time to herself as I went to do farm chores outside. The hour I spent outside seemed to drag on like it was three hours. When I was inside with Emily the clock just seemed to turn twice as fast as it was actually going.

Chapter 14

The Comparison

This would be a good time to explain the difference that I experienced now compared to when my daughter was born 17 years ago. With Emily we are now at 39 weeks and our baby boy was ready to be delivered.

The pregnancy I went through with Clare was much different. We had the birthing center booked and our bags were packed. We were just waiting on our daughter to let us know that she was ready to be delivered.

In our state the birthing center could only deliver up to two weeks after the due date. Seeing as how Clare and the first midwife, at the birthing center, just randomly picked the due date; this had some serious consequences.

It was the hottest part of summer and the peak of storm season. I felt that the constant barometric pressure changes would bring on Clare's labor, but it never did. We were in the final week that we were allowed to deliver the baby at the birthing center and there wasn't even a sign of labor yet.

Remember earlier when I said that we had a new midwife that took over Clare's care? She wasn't very helpful through this process. Our birthing deadline was approaching fast and we were about to lose the opportunity to deliver at the birthing center.

Where would this leave us, if the birthing center would no longer let us into their office to birth our baby? They didn't give us a good answer, or offer any advice on how to bring on labor faster as this deadline was approaching.

There was a hurricane brewing and we were preparing to have it hit just north of our home, in the last stages of Clare's pregnancy. We were making preparations by boarding up the windows, doors and tying anything down that would fly away. This seemed to put extra strain on Clare. I was pretty sure that my daughter would be born anytime now or when this storm hit landfall.

Clare had spoken to the birth center. She told them that if anything was to happen, she would get there as soon as she could. They agreed that they would work with us as we were only days away from losing their care.

Maybe it was a sign from above that we had made bad choices in life, or the heavens were angry at us for some reason? That hurricane turned at the last minute and it came right over top of our home. The pressure changed as the winds surged, you could feel your ears popping! The barometric pressure was dropping fast and that didn't bring on even a single contraction. My daughter just wasn't ready to come out yet.

After the water stopped poring through our ceilings and the house stopped shaking, I unbolted the door to walk out and see that we now lived in a disaster zone. This wasn't the beautiful home that we once lived in, it looked like a picture from a horror movie and I was the main character. Everything was leveled for as far as I could see. We had just gone through one of the worst events of our lives.

The house flooded with water and all the shingles were gone from the roof. There was not any safe place in there for us anymore. There was no telephone signal and the roads were all blocked with downed trees, poles and powerlines. We had no way to contact the birth center if we wanted to. With our house destroyed we had nowhere to even stay that was safe for Clare and my daughter.

The only place that we had to stay now was an old RV that was on the property. The inside of it was semi dry and the roof only leaked in a few places. There was no running water or power services to speak of. There weren't even power poles left standing. This was our only option as the home that we were just in was now uninhabitable.

It took two full days until FEMA cleared the roads enough that the National Guard let us out to the interstate. Our local hospital was destroyed and there was no one to call for help.

When we finally made it to the birthing center, they were closed and unavailable. We had limited phone service, but were able to get a call into them. The midwife came to meet us.

We had told the midwife what happened to us. There really wasn't very much compassion from her on our new crappy situation. We were not looking for pity or anything other than to have this baby in their birthing center. Her response was that we were now a day past the two-week deadline and were beyond the date that they could offer us services. We would no longer be able to deliver at their center.

Just like that, we no longer had a place to deliver our baby. The $5500 dollars that we had spent was gone and so was our home. Along with everything that we had worked so hard for.

The midwife did mention that since we didn't use the center, there would be a small refund due back to us. After they figured out all of the billable hours and expenses that we incurred for the up-to-date tests and exams. We didn't need a refund! We needed a place to have our daughter.

Fast forward a little: Clare did manage to get us a refund from the birthing center. ONE HUNDRED DOLLARS was the refund for not using their facility and that took months to actually receive.

I can't stress enough, that the hurricane wasn't the reason we couldn't use their services. It wasn't that the baby wasn't ready to come out yet. It sure wasn't due to anything that we did in the process. We timed out of their care because the midwife and Clare picked and agreed on a due date from the last time Clare took a birth control pill. They had no way of verifying when Clare's last period was, or the actual conception date.

I remember the moment when my daughter was made, I just didn't remember what day or even week it was. Clare didn't know because she never kept track of anything. She just guessed and in turn the midwife just guessed also. We were now suffering the consequences of this mistake.

We also didn't end up with the midwife we were happy with and we signed up with. At the end we had the fill in midwife, that knew nothing about Clare's pregnancy or her in general. All that she knew was what she read on the chart.

The midwife did offer to escort us to the hospital and stay with us throughout the labor. We agreed on this as we needed someone to help guide us through this situation. This is the point where things turned for the worse.

When we arrived at the hospital, I will never forget, we had to wait for the midwife to finish smoking her cigarette before we went inside. Clare and I had been through enough over the past several days and really didn't need her shenanigans. I was young and didn't know any better, or I would have never even had her take us to that hospital.

As we walked up to the emergency room doors and they opened, I could feel the rush of air pushing on my face. It felt like the air was telling me to turn around and leave. We didn't leave, we headed inside. The intake lady was doing an interview with us and was confused as to why we were there.

Clare showed no signs of labor, even her water hadn't broken. The only thing that the midwife could tell the lady at the intake desk, was that she wasn't legally allowed to deliver our baby anymore.

If anyone was confused, I was. How did we even end up here to begin with? Seems like when you start to have things figured out, life puts more pressure on you to see how much you can take. I was running out of energy quick.

They didn't admit us to the ER, they couldn't. There was no emergency! The baby wasn't ready to be born yet and still needed more time inside of Clare.

We were given instructions on how to get to the maternity ward and sent up the elevator. As we made our way down the hall, the lady there greeted us at the door to let us in. We went to what looked to be the nurse area. The nurses were asking Clare and I questions as to why we were there? They wanted to know who our doctor was and so on. They were confused as to why we had come there in the first place. I was confused also. We were only there for the midwife to transfer care and the hospital didn't want us.

The midwife tried to explain that she was our care provider, but she could no longer care for us. The hospital asked if Clare was in labor or having any symptoms and the answer was no. They then had to consult with the doctor on duty to see what they could even do with us.

The midwife offered no help toward anything. She was really just there to eventually send us a bill for the hospital drop off. The hospital didn't recognize her practice or even who she was. They wouldn't allow her to stay in the maternity ward with us. We were once again on our own and had no one to lean on.

After a talk with the resident doctor, he asked what we wanted to do? We didn't know what to do. We expressed to him that we were two weeks past the due date and were not sure how to handle this now that we had no care provider.

He eventually had us admitted to a room for observation. It was a tiny exam room and there was barely enough room for me and one nurse in there.

At this point we were now in the care of a hospital and no longer had any say as to the natural birth we were supposed to have.

It was now 9:00 in the morning. The nurse hooked Clare up to an IV bag. They put monitors on her finger and were checking her blood pressure.

The doctor seemed pretty angry that we came into the hospital without an appointment and without having our own physician. There weren't any other words spoken from him after he looked over Clare's vitals.

Now Clare wasn't having any signs of labor or anything when we arrived. Her water never even broke. It was all a matter of the birth center cutting their care from us that put Clare in that hospital bed.

The Nurse was adding things to the IV bag and was in and out of the room a lot. Within an hour or so they stated that Clare wasn't progressing. They broke her water for her. In went that screw in monitor into the baby's head and they were adding more things to the IV bag.

Around about 11:00AM the pain started to set in and Clare was having contractions. She asked them if she could have something for the pain and they declined. They told her that it was too late for an epidural.

By this point I could see that they had started the contractions by whatever they put in the IV bag. These people were not messing around. I was watching the monitors as there was nothing else for me to do besides holding Clare's hand.

Coming up on 12:00 noon now, they stated that she still wasn't progressing fast enough. Clare was in pain as the contractions came on so fast and hard. She was gripping my hand tighter and tighter as her pelvis was twisting in pain.

The doctor came back in at 12:30PM. He told Clare that she just wasn't progressing fast enough and that he could offer her a cesarian. He stated that this would relieve her pain. His second option was that, she could wait until he got back from lunch at 3:30PM and see how things were progressing then.

The stress that we were under over being homeless, losing everything, along with the lack of sleep and defeat pushed Clare to want to give up. They left the room to let us talk about it and I was against it. I wanted to have the baby as naturally as possible, but Clare didn't want to do it anymore. The doctor's offer of it all being over in thirty minutes pushed Clare to the breaking point. She just wanted it over with.

The nurse came back in to emphasize that the doctor would be going to lunch if she didn't want the cesarian. Then just like that, their slick ways of being decent salesmen, pushed Clare into saying "just do it". My say was now overruled by her word that she gave to the nurse to just get this over with.

I was asked to leave the room as three extra nurses came in to prep Clare for surgery. I looked at Clare one last time, like it would be the last time I saw her as I stood in the doorway. The flock of nurses pulled her gown back, one was using a razor to shave her stomach just above her pubic area and the other was preparing to remove her from the monitors.

I was then escorted by a staff member down the hall and outside of the maternity ward. This was the last time that I was able to see Clare. They were taking her to surgery and I was not allowed to be with her.

Chapter 15

Hello Labor Day

Emily laughed at first, like the cramps were nothing. "They are no worse than light period cramps" she was telling me; while we sat at the computer together to finish some last-minute work. She was bouncing on her yoga ball and I was just blasting away on the keyboard. I had this feeling that once the cramps began to get worse, I would not be able to get much done. Finishing up my work now was a must.

Emily pulled up a page on the internet that let you log your contractions. I had the job of pushing the button on the mouse when she said go and then I had to press it again when the contraction was over. This was creating what looked to be a spread sheet of how long they were and the time in between the contractions.

Lasting from thirty seconds to one minute and being five minutes apart, this wasn't a big concern to her. The more she bounced on the yoga ball the faster they would get. When she wanted them to drag out longer, she would walk around the house and they became further apart.

When we started this contraction counter it was still daylight out. Now it was coming up on 9:30 in the evening. This baby was not ready to come out anytime soon from the looks of it. The contractions were really far apart and Emily was not in very much pain up until now.

Asking her when we should call the midwife, she said that we weren't even close to that point yet. There is another factor that came into play here; if we did call the midwife, she would have started the ticking clock on us. This would mean that she would consistently be messaging Emily to check on her. Emily did not want her phone even turned on; let alone have to message the midwife updates. Knowing that we had a set of wishes we wanted honored, it was easier for us to keep control of the labor and not turn it over quite yet.

Drinking lots of water and having to pee constantly, I figured that I would sneak in a nap while Emily was in the bathroom. I must have dosed off about 10:30 Saturday evening and Emily let me sleep. This was the last sleep I would be getting though. At 11:30PM, just one hour into my power nap, I was awakened to what felt like I was being shaken to death. Now in reality she was just trying to get my attention, but when your knocked out you never know what's happening when you wake up and you're still asleep.

This was it, I figured that she was ready to deliver our son and we would be back to bed. What happened in that hour I was asleep was pretty crazy! Emily wasn't asleep next to me; she was laboring the whole time. The position she was laying in was bringing the contractions on harder and faster. It was now time that she needed me and I had to snap out of my dream state.

Her voice had grown deeper now and she was starting to let out her emotions. This baby was coming now and there was no turning back. I was rubbing Emily's arms trying to comfort her. That didn't work. Then I spoke to her gently and kindly trying to comfort her. That wasn't working either!

I hit the internet one last time to try and find some answers; to both bring on the labor faster and ease the pain. There was so much information it was hard to decipher what was good and what would work for us.

Finding a short list of pressure points that both bring on labor and help the process along, I went for it. I drew a little map of where they were supposed to be on a small note card and ran back into the room.

Pulling Emily toward the edge of the bed, I found the two points that were on her lower back. I pressed my thumbs into the little hollow, it's about an inch to the side, just off the top of where her butt crack ends into her back. She started to make a sound; I must have been in the right spot. Putting more pressure on her I could feel her body start to loosen. Pushing harder until it felt like my thumbs fell asleep. I eased back off and gave her a minute.

Next there was a spot on the inside of her lower legs, just above the ankles. I did the same thing here as she was pushing through another contraction. Repeating over and over, I alternated where I would push, to not aggravate Emily in any way. The contractions were starting to set in pretty hard now and they were more frequent.

She had to get out of the bed she said. I helped her off the tall platform bed we were in, walked her to the bathroom and she wanted to try the shower. I helped her peel off her clothes and in she went. The hot water started to slow the contractions and she was in euphoria over it.

It's 12:00AM now, Hello Sunday! Our son just managed to hang in there for 23.5 hours and didn't seem to want out yet. The best part of this was that it was Sunday the day of rest. Well, that really wasn't the case for this Sunday, maybe next Sunday. Emily was now sitting on the shower floor and the water was just running down her body. She seemed to enjoy the relief it offered and her contractions were now further apart.

We knew from the time that we hired the midwife that most woman preferred a water birth over any other style. The midwife offered for us to use the inflatable tub she has available. While that seemed ok, we had an old farm house that was pretty well equipped already.

Several years ago, when I remodeled the spare bathroom on the far side of the house, I installed a *copper* clawfoot tub. At the time I really didn't have a reason for wanting that tub. I just had a feeling it would be needed some day. The room has barely ever been used and it just sits there collecting dust. Good thing I cleaned it really well last night.

While Emily was burning through all the hot water in the shower, I set the tub on lukewarm and let it start to fill. I threw a giant pot on the stove with water and left it to boil. Back to the shower I went to hold Emily's hand and make sure she was ok. This would be one of the last breaks I would have for the next several hours.

Off to make sure that boiling water made it into the tub. I poured it in and set the pot back on the stove for round two. This tub was going to need 50 plus gallons to get started and the water was barely room temperature.

This evening, the temperature outside had dropped and we had to turn the heat on in the house. The floors were ice cold and I was having trouble keeping the house a comfortable temperature for Emily. Her hormones were raging and the swings went from too hot to too cold in what seemed to be seconds.

I ran back in and shut off the tub in hopes that the hot water heater would eventually catch up. Then I darted back to help Emily out of the shower. Drying her off, I could see the fluids that once filled her belly to protect the baby were all but gone. As I ran my hand over her stomach, all I could feel was the outline of my son.

Taking her back to the bed, I wanted to hear his heart again. I had tried to use the stethoscope we had in the birthing kit, but that was a bust. I moved my ear around on her stomach until I came to her lower left side and there it was. I could feel the strong fast beat of my son's heart.

Emily needed me to help her but she didn't know how. I placed my hands on her lower back and pushed. This was what she needed. I tried rubbing her upper back but that just aggravated her, so I stuck to the lower back. When I would try and let up the pressure, she would tell me to put them back and that's what I did.

Wanting to give her some relief, we had a heating pad with the birthing kit. I ran to get that and plugged it in. Now it took a little while to heat up, but once it did, I wrapped it on her back and she started to feel a slight bit of relief. Still pushing on her, while the pad was warming her, it seemed to work for an hour or so.

Her contractions were now building again and were between one and two minutes apart. This was making it very difficult for me to catch a break. As the contraction would come on, I would have to push on her back. Only letting up after the contraction went away. This gave me roughly one to two minutes to get that tub turned back on and try to go to the bathroom.

I didn't really get to go, even though my belly was rumbling and I needed to. Every time I went to sit on the toilet, she would scream for me and up I would go right back to her. I've learned through this process that when the labor starts there is no break. There is no time to even go to the bathroom. Your attention is now one hundred percent focused on mom and baby.

At this point there was nowhere that Emily could lay or sit that was comfortable. Even the magic of that shower had worn off and she was in pain. The walk to the other side of the house seemed pretty easy, until we had to stop in the kitchen for another contraction that bent her over the counter. I was pushing on her lower back and could feel the pain radiating through her.

Emily wasn't screaming in pain; it was more of a dry crying mixed with the howl of a wolf. The peaceful music that filled the house was now being muffled by her voice. I was helpless, all I wanted to do was take away her pain, but I didn't know how. I attempted an icepack from the freezer, but this offered no relief at all. It would seem that the forty or so more steps required, to get to the other side of the house, would take thirty minutes to accomplish.

The tub was now full and I reached over to turn the water off. Back to the kitchen to grab Emily and we were off. She was shuffling across the old wood floor on her way to the next destination on the list of stops. She sat down on the toilet before getting into the tub. I used a flashlight to look between her legs and I couldn't see any change. The baby's head wasn't out and everything looked normal. She urinated and there was no blood and no extra fluids. I felt that we were getting close, but now I felt defeated.

Wrapping her arms around my neck I helped her up. She leaned into me, stretching her back out and was feeling relief. The relief was only temporary as the next contraction set in. She howled in my ear letting the pain out and pulled fresh air in to help ease the contraction. Contractions were now a minute apart and there was no slowing this process down. Emily was going to have this baby soon.

Still wrapped around me she picked her right leg up over the lip on the tub into water. I helped her with the other leg to keep her from losing balance. Lowering my body down as she was still wrapped around my neck, she was in the water now. While she was trying to find a comfortable position, I ran to the kitchen to refill her drinking water tumbler. She was belting out come back and off I went. I was needed to push on her back while she was in the water.

Leaning in and under the water was getting pretty exhausting to me. Turning the shower wand on full hot, I used it to massage her lower back and she closed her eyes as it eased the pain. I was onto something here. Using a circular motion, I went up and down her back until her howls subsided. Then I would turn the water off to give it a minute break.

This went on for an hour or so and she needed to try a new position now. Helping her out of the warm water she was shivering, but her body was plenty warm. The shivers were coming from the pain that Emily was experiencing.

I helped her to the bed that was just outside of the bathroom door and ran to get her more blankets. As prepared as I was, I had plenty of towels, but no extra blankets in that room. Returning as fast as I could, less than forty-five seconds, I beat the next contraction. I started to wrap her tight in several of them. I laid next to her and rubbed up and down her body to bring heat into her. It was at this time that I wondered if our son could feel everything that she was feeling? Or if he would ever remember any of this pain?

The pain that she was feeling set in to the point where she told me to get the throw up bag. Boy am I glad that we had a twenty pack of them, because we were about to need them. *Tip! Do NOT cheap out on these things. Get as many as you can afford, you will need them.* I started opening up the bags out of the twenty pack Emily bought and sitting them everywhere. They were within arm's reach at all times.

It wasn't but twenty minutes later and well, she was right, she needed a throw up bag. I had no idea she was so hydrated at this point. She sure filled the first one up, then the second and third one as well. This happened several times throughout the night as the pain worsened. If I never see her do that again I will be grateful.

For the next several hours I tried everything to make Emily comfortable, and nothing worked. I had her bouncing on the yoga ball and that did nothing. I made her get on her knees, on the bed and used a wedge under her to prop her up, that did nothing. The only thing that even seemed to work was her laying on her left side. I placed a pillow between her legs and that took away some of the pressure, but I was still pushing on her back for one minute on and one minute off, for the last several hours.

You would think time would stand still while this was happening and that is not the case at all. The arms on the clock were flying around. The cuckoo clock was blurting out the time in 30-minute intervals for us from the living room. I got to the point that I was laying next to her pushing on her and I started to fall asleep. Emily caught onto that maneuver I tried and woke me right back up.

This went on for hours throughout the early Sunday morning. The sun was now coming up and Emily had made it to morning. We weren't going to have my son in the cover of darkness, he would now be born as the sun was rising, or so I thought he would.

Emily had so much pressure on her lower half that she wanted to walk around. We had been in and out of the tub over the past several hours. This process just seemed like it would never end. Walking through the house, the contractions were getting worse and closer together. She said she had to go to the bathroom and it wasn't going to wait.

We stopped in the master bathroom. As she was peeing, I was looking with a flashlight between her legs. She was swollen down there now and everything was bulging. I could tell that we were getting very close now. I assured Emily that it wouldn't be long. As she sat there her bowels were emptying and I had to leave for that moment. I went to lay on the bed and as soon as I hit the pillow, she screamed my name again. I tried to just lay there, but nope, she screamed again and up I went. Back into the room to examine what had made its way out of her before she flushed. Now a man can deal with a lot, but examining your wife's poop is pushing it.

I wiped her back side and helped her into the shower. I didn't want any cross contamination to get on my baby boy. Rubbing her down with soap and the hot water, she was taking in the thirty seconds of freedom she had from the contractions.

This shower lasted quite some time and the hot water was about to be cold again. Emily was laying on the shower floor and I was holding her hand. This was the moment that she warned me about when we started this journey. She told me that there was going to be a point where she wants to give up all together. That would be the starting point for me to encourage her further along. I did this for a long while and we made a deal. If we got to 9:00AM and nothing was progressing that we would call the midwife for additional support.

The hot water was now a thing of the past and I needed to get Emily back up off the shower floor. She wrapped her arms around my neck and I pulled her up out of there. Drying her off she was leaning on the sink in agony. She was in the final stretch. The howls were coming out just as loud, but they now had a mixture of her tiredness haunting them. I was defeated myself. There was no easy fix I could offer her. I felt like I had failed and let my family down.

I made that call at 9:22AM on Emily's phone. I was still pushing on her back and she was howling at the window, as she was laying sideways on the bed. The midwife answered after about 9 or so rings. I was sure that it would have gone to voicemail, but she answered.

This was the only time through this whole process that Emily would call her for anything. I had to handle the call as the howls were full term now and Emily couldn't speak anymore.

The midwife asked how long the labor had been going on and just some basic questions. I had it on speaker so that she could hear Emily's howls and screams to time the contractions. This was the first time that Emily felt vulnerable and had to ask for help this whole pregnancy.

Chapter 16

At Home Delivery

Transition, is what they call it when you reach the peak. It's the final stage of labor and Emily had made it to this point on her own. Just before I called the midwife I did feel between Emily's legs and I could feel the baby's head. She had finally made the progress that she needed and it was ok now that we made that call for help.

The midwife stayed on the phone as she was on the road traveling to us. She also dispatched her assistant, Laura, who was closer to us and could arrive sooner. Should we have given them a heads up that Emily was this far along? Perhaps, but the fact is that this is how Emily wanted to do this. I'm her husband and her rock, so we stuck to the plan.

Not even an hour later there was a text that came through, she was 3 minutes out. I would need to leave

Emily for just a minute to let Laura in, but Emily wouldn't let me leave her side. I was still pushing and rubbing her lower back, that's what she needed. The breathing techniques that were coming through the phone couldn't help Emily. She couldn't hear them over her howls.

It was 10:10AM and Laura had arrived. I waited until the last contraction ended and ran to unlock the door to let her in. Stepping out of her car; she was then running toward the door. In my lack of sleep delirium, all that I could see was what appeared to be an angel running at me. I opened the door for her and in she went. She knew where to go as she followed the sounds of Emily's howls.

The backup that we needed had just arrived. There was a calm that came over me. Laura, in her bare feet and scrubs, jumped up on the bed and went to work. She wasted no time at all. With the midwife just a few minutes away she hung up the phone while Laura worked. Leaning over the side of the bed, I was holding Emily's hand as Laura put her into position. She put her on her knees and piled pillows under her stomach and breasts.

Emily's howls grew even louder now and she was full on screaming. She screamed that it hurt so bad and I could feel her pain radiating into my heart through her hand. Emily was getting defeated and she was already through the hardest part. Laura grabbed her hips and started working them like she was going to wiggle the baby out of there. Emily was dehydrated at this point from not being able to drink, so I ran to the kitchen to make her a vitamin and mineral smoothie.

Walking back into the room, I had to stop for a minute and gaze at the sight I saw. It was my wife, having her hips worked by our new angel and it about brought tears to my eyes. Emily's whole body was moving side to side and back and forth, as Laura swayed with her. This baby would have no choice but to wiggle out now or he would have a full body workout before being born.

Emily was still in pain, but knowing that Laura was there supporting and teaching her to breathe was just what she needed. I made Emily drink through a straw and start to add fluids back into her. This was replacing the fluids that she lost vomiting throughout the night. She was drinking water all night and morning, but there is no replacement for the salt and sugar that she needed.

Twenty minutes into Laura coaching Emily and the midwife arrived. I ran to the door to greet her; she had a couple suitcases with her that contained her supplies. In she came and she knew right were to go. She just followed the howls and moans.

At this point my adrenaline started to kick back in and that tiredness I felt went away. The dogs were going crazy and I had to go lock them outside. I ran back in to not miss a moment of the labor.

This was the first time that the baby would have his heart rate checked by the doppler. The midwife had set up office and she was going to work charting. Laura was still breathing with Emily moving her out of transition to use the fetal ejection reflex.

Now at this point, when the professionals were on the scene, nothing I could say mattered anymore and I was shut out. Even though they couldn't get an answer from Emily, they refused to listen to me. Even though I was there for this whole event.

The midwife wanted to do a cervical exam at this point, but it was too late. The baby was too close and we didn't want her to introduce any bacteria into Emily. That was something that we decided on before the labor even started.

After about ten minutes of charting and Laura still working Emily's hips, Emily needed to go to the bathroom. The bathroom that Emily needed to use was across the house, with the tub. The midwife did another check with the doppler to chart the baby's heart rate first.

Emily wiggled herself to the end of the bed and off her and Laura went. They started to make their way to that room. No sooner did Emily try and sit on the toilet and my sons head was out up to his ears. I could see it sticking out about 2.5 inches past her labia. Emily didn't have to pee after all, she was delivering our son.

Laura belted out "partial", yelling to the midwife, and the midwife came right away.

Helping Emily into the tub was the next move. We made sure we didn't bump his head on the rim of the tub as Emily entered the lukewarm water. The midwife told Emily, you can reach down and feel your son's head, and that she did. The dry howls were now slightly replaced with what could only be described as howls of pure joy.

Emily had already done all the hard work on her own. She just needed the extra support from the midwife and Laura to make the final delivery. This was something new to Emily and she needed to know that she had done everything right.

The breathing was what mattered at this point. Emily never once tried to push our son out. She let mother nature do all the work. She just endured the pain throughout the process. The baby was coming out and all the hard work that went on for the last two days was coming to a close.

Emily found the best position to be in was on her knees in the tub. This would help the baby come out easier. She just felt the baby's head and this was the home stretch. During one of the contractions the baby started to retract and was being pulled back inside of Emily. She lifted her right leg up and placed her foot flat on the bottom of the tub. This stopped that and the baby started to move in the right direction again.

That bath water was cooling off too fast and I needed to warm her up. I used the shower wand again and set it to HOT! I started working her lower back like I did for the last twelve hours. The ladies swore it wouldn't help now, but Emily wouldn't let me stop. She needed that heat on her to ease the last few contractions.

Within a few minutes and a howl that I will never forget, the baby's head was out. The midwife was coaching Emily on how to bring him out. Her belly was so big her short arms were having trouble reaching the baby's shoulders. Emily asked for help and the midwife released the cord that was holding him back. She gave him a nudge to release his broad shoulders.

With a few more deep breaths, my son passed the rest of his body through the birth canal and he was free. I could see him floating under the water in his mom's hands. It was so beautiful to see! Emily's emotions filled the room and there was nothing but love in the air.

This made the last two days worth every minute that Emily and I did this together. Emily had now achieved an assisted home birth in forty-five minutes time. Only forty-five minutes in the midwife's care and my baby was born. This made the whole experience worth it to Emily and I. We didn't have to have a whole house full of strangers and we were left to do it on Emily's terms.

I can't express enough that you need to have a plan and you need to hire the professionals. Even if you don't use them, or you only use them at the last minute. You still have them there for you if you need them. I can handle a lot on the farm, from delivering to reviving cattle and other animals. On delivery day, I was sure glad that we had a support system in place and it wasn't just me.

What I learned through this, is that it didn't matter whether we were to have a boy or a girl. I didn't care what he or she would look like, or even if they had not enough or too many fingers or toes. I knew one thing for sure. I made this baby and it was my gift from above. Before we knew we were pregnant, I had prayed, and asked for everything that I wanted in a child. Then I prayed and asked for everything that I didn't want in a child.

Take the way I did this for what it's worth to you. I knew what I wanted in a child before I made the little angel. But I also know that you get what you can handle in life and well, I can handle a whole lot! No matter what I was gifted in a child, I knew one thing, I already loved him or her no matter what I was given!

This child was mine and Emily's, we wanted him. The thing is that there are always variables that you can't account for. You try to make the right choices up front and with good intentions. When life's plan for you changes, you will have to be ready to take what's coming your way.

When the doctors delivered Clare's baby by cesarian, I lost the opportunity to be a part of everything like I just experienced with Emily. I do not wish that loss on anyone.

I do not have a great birth story that I can tell you with the hospital birth. It was not a great story in any way. I missed out on being there when Clare needed me the most. A doctor took my place. I never had the chance to watch my daughter be born into this world. I never had the bonding experience like the one that I'm about to share with you. I never had the ability to share my love with Clare as the baby was removed from her. I don't ever want to go through that again for any reason. It's my wish that no one else will either.

The next part for Emily and I was life changing. Still on her knees in the tub, I have stopped running hot water on her. The pain was now gone! The only thing that filled the room now was love and tears of happiness.

Emily was crying real tears this time and they were tears of love. She had just done what could seem to be impossible to some. She delivered her own child, in her own tub at her home. This was exhilarating and slightly overwhelming to her. Her emotions couldn't be held back now, as her heart released a waterfall of joy that blanketed our newborn baby son.

My son was held tight to Emily's chest and the midwife gave them a minute to bond. I was holding his little body with my hand and it was a magical moment. He grunted slightly and I knew he was ok; he had just tried to take his first breath in his new home. How beautiful this was to me!

The midwife and Laura moved me back so that they could work now. They were checking his lungs and removing any fluid from his airway. It was only seconds later that he started to cry. This made it official, my baby boy was here to stay.

Emily stayed in the tub for a short while. We covered him with a towel to keep him warm in the water, as he was pressed to Emily's chest. Not very long later the placenta started to deliver itself. Emily explained that they were just cramps, nothing like the labor pains. In just a few cramps the placenta fell into the tub. This all took place so fast that I almost missed it! I was too distracted staring at my baby boy.

The placenta was placed in a bowl and we transferred Emily to the bed. There was nothing more reassuring than Emily being able to stand up and walk herself to the bed. The only help she needed was getting over the lip of the tub and on to steady ground. This was such a great experience and I'm glad that I was able to be present for this.

Emily was moving around to find her comfortable spot in bed, while the midwife was just at the end of the bed. I laid there with Emily and my son for a few minutes to let him know who I was. The midwife left to finish her charting and then Laura gave us some time to be alone.

This experience is one that can't be replaced by a birth center or other institution. The baby was just born and now you're resting in your own bed, no traveling or deadlines to leave. Emily just had our baby and she is now resting fifteen feet from where the baby was born. This is how every birth should be.

My son was already getting familiar with the new territory. He was searching for the nipple already and wanted his colostrum. He had no pain medicine or drugs in his system to slow him down. He was ready to begin his new life as our son.

This experience was the polar opposite with my daughter. Clare had been put under anesthesia. I didn't see her again, until they wheeled her into her new recovery room at the hospital. I just missed the first hour of my daughter's life and there was no getting that time back. I didn't get to hear her first breath being taken. I surely didn't get to congratulate Clare on making a beautiful baby girl. All that I had to keep me company was my worries and tears while I tried to keep it together in the waiting room.

After Clare was settled into her recovery room, they invited me in. A nurse then rolled my daughter into the room. This would be the actual first time that I had the chance to put my hands on my newborn daughter.

Now Clare was unconscious and they had her on a morphine drip. The first time I actually had the chance to hold my daughter, her mom was unconscious and I just held her tight in her already swaddled hospital blanket. I only knew she was a girl from the tag that they put on her rolling crib, and the word of the nurse that wouldn't let me hold her in the waiting room.

This was not an ideal situation to me. I knew that my daughter was hungry by now and Clare was not available for this task. I unwrapped my daughter from the swaddle and pulled Clare's hospital gown to the other side over her arm. I was in control now and wanted to be sure that she received her colostrum.

As I was placing her on her mom's chest, I noticed that her foot was cut. I brought the nurse in and they explained that must have been done in surgery and it would be ok. This angered me, now my brand-new baby was not only cut from her mother's womb, but was also physically cut.

It took me hours to get my daughter to latch onto Clare. I was persistent and wouldn't give up. Clare woke up here and there, but would only mumble. She was out of it and had no idea where she even was.

This experience has left scars on my heart that can't be removed. To be so helpless in a situation and have no control, is something I hope no one has to ever experience. I missed out on cutting the cord, baby's first cry and the bonding experience that I just had with my son.

Emily, on the other hand, was alert and seemed to have a whole second wind after her and my son slept for about thirty minutes. The midwife came back into the room and it was now time to take some measurements and vitals from the baby.

I only had one more task to do and I kind of blew it. It was my job to cut the cord. You would think that this was easy and I'm sure that it is. Well, as part of the birth kit, we bought a stainless-steel cord cutter. As with all things you buy these days, they were junk. The midwife had the cord pinched off real close to the baby and all I had to do was snip. I opened the cutters and tried to snip, but the cutters were struggling. Either that, or the kids' cord was made of steel, we are still not sure.

The thought had crossed my mind to just run out to our barn and grab the electrical cable cutters I have; them things will cut anything. Emily wouldn't go for that, so I just squeezed a little harder and sure enough they cut right through. Finally, I was able to cut the cord of one of my children. This was a great feeling and made me very proud. I was the one that was able to remove my son's lifeline that kept him safe for the last ten months.

The rest of the home birth experience was pretty great. I was off to heat up the soup and potatoes I made Emily yesterday. She would need the energy and nutrition to keep her going. It's only just after high noon and we were back to our normal life like nothing had even happened.

The duties that still needed taking care of Laura and the midwife were undertaking. Laura was cleaning up the piles of towels we had used and washing down the tub for us. She even went as far to do a load of laundry too. The midwife was weighing the baby checking his length and girth.

Now Emily had to use the bathroom and the midwife helped her to the edge of the bed and checked her vitals. Emily's heart rate was still slightly high so she rested for a moment. Then they headed to the toilet. The midwife showed Emily how to use a post-partum water bottle to clean herself out after urination. She was very helpful with advice on how to stay clean and heal.

After Emily came back to the bed, the midwife performed a vaginal inspection to be sure that there was no major bleeding. Sure enough, Emily had done so well there were no major problems to speak of. She didn't need an episiotomy during labor and everything looked as though it would heal up nicely. With only small tears on the inside of the labia; they didn't need stitches or surgery. We attributed this to not pushing and letting the baby come out when he was ready. This was a big deal to Emily as she could heal faster. Emily felt no pain from the small tears and had an awesome recovery.

Now with Clare in the hospital, she didn't have a vaginal birth. Therefore, I had nothing to compare this home birth with. Clare had sutures and dressing on her stomach. She couldn't have the baby on top of her from the pain in her stomach after the cesarian.

The whole process after the birth of my son was wrapped up pretty quick. Emily was well on her way to breastfeeding my son. They were wrapped up in the blankets together in our bed. The midwife and Laura stayed for another hour or so to make sure that everything was going ok with Emily, then they left.

It made Emily very happy to know that from the time we called them and they arrived, the baby was out in forty-five minutes. After the baby was born, they were only here for a little over three hours. Emily was ecstatic that we could go back to our life now and there wasn't anyone to entertain or look after. It was just me, Emily and my son as a family. We were ready to start a new chapter in our life.

Chapter 17
Dad Acting As Mom

It's been four hours since my beautiful little son came into this world. Now the work starts all over again. Emily's busy with making sure that he gets plenty of nutrition and takes in all the colostrum she can produce. They have bonded already and my son is working her nipple like an old pro. I know that he had a very long journey to get here, but he was built with the instincts to latch on and feed himself.

Emily has been through so much in the last 43.5 hours and I would have thought that she needed a nap. Dozing off for just a few minutes, the rush of adrenaline she received from now holding our son in her arms, was better than any cup of coffee or shot of sugar. She wasn't ready to sleep. The four hours of sleep that she had a couple of days ago was still fueling her through this entire process.

The hardest part of the process is that after she was settled in and nursing our son, there were still strangers in our home. That could make a woman somewhat uncomfortable.

Now she knew that I was handling everything, but the fact that she still felt the need to be helpful never passed. This is where as a dad, it is our job to step up to the plate and just take over. I had to run my household now. Emily had a new full-time job and it was recovering and resting. Along with being there to feed our son, as he was hungry.

Making sure that I had the opportunity to lay with them for a little while so that our son could bond with me, was an essential part of the process also. Emily needed to refuel and the first thing she ate was a bowl of sweet potatoes, then she washed that down with a small amount of veggie soup. To keep her going I made her a fresh vitamin and mineral juice smoothie. This would give her the power she needed to get my son his colostrum.

I kept on top of her to keep drinking water as well. After throwing up several times early this morning, this led to her fluid levels being very low. The best part is that the baby is here now, we are at our home and never had to go anywhere.

The process was not nearly the same with my daughter and Clare though. The hospital had discharged us on the fourth morning after my daughter was born. The bad part about this was, that we were now homeless and had no where safe to go. Before leaving the hospital, I had called every hotel in a hundred-mile radius. There was only one room left available. This hotel was about 2.5 hours north of the hospital. I booked the room and off we went.

Packing our small diaper bag, the nurse came in and put Clare in a wheel chair and down the elevator we went. They would only release us if we had a car seat in the car, which we did. Out the same double doors that I walked into four days ago we went. I pulled the car around and the nurse helped Clare out of the wheel chair. I loaded our bag in the trunk, seat belted the car seat in and helped Clare into the back seat.

Now I'm not an expert here, but after the major surgery, was she supposed to be in so much pain? Clare couldn't barely walk. The two steps it took to get into the car, she was teared up and holding her stomach like it was falling out she claimed.

Along our journey to the hotel, every time I would hit a bump in the road, Clare would grunt in pain. I could see her tearing up in my rear-view mirror. The two-and-a-half-hour trip seemed like it took days to get there. There was no room service at the hotel, I can't even remember eating anything that evening. As soon as we were settled into the room, Clare passed out.

It was my job to be sure that my daughter got latched on and ate that night. This was a daunting task as Clare was passed out from her pain pills. I had to stay up all night with my newborn. I made her eat several times throughout the night. Clare's milk wasn't coming in very strong, but it was enough to satisfy my daughters little tummy so she could sleep for a little while.

As the sun rose that morning, I was looking out the window asking what I did wrong in life to deserve what I was going through. Why did I get picked for this lousy journey? Why couldn't I just have what we planned originally to happen come true and this all end?

Well, I didn't get an answer that day and I didn't get that answer for many years to come. I only received what I asked for when I actually asked for it, not just hoped for it. The experience with Clare changed me. It changed my outlook on life and made me believe that you get given what you can handle in life.

The experience that I just had with Emily was what I wanted the first time; I just wasn't ready for that experience 17 years ago. I had to find out what hard times were, so that I could appreciate the good times when they came.

Leaving the hotel that day, we had nowhere to go. I pointed the car south and headed back to the disaster zone. As we pulled off the interstate exit, all I could see was sadness and pain. The losses that affected, not just us, but the rest of the town was pretty real now. When you're in it, it's one thing, but coming back to it after you have left is another. A few curves of the road and we were back to our new home from this point on.

I backed the car in the driveway and I carried our bag and the baby carrier to the now flooded out RV. The water tank in it had leaked and it flooded the floor to top off the situation. Guess the hurricane had damaged it more than I originally noticed.

I helped Clare inside, we were now running on a generator and had AC at least. There was no way to bathe or keep Clare's incision clean other than bottled water and paper towels. I know that this was about the worse case scenario after having major surgery, but this is what we were willed in life and we had to deal with it.

Needless to say, I don't have anything positive to say about the experience after the hospital, so I will just leave it at this. My daughter was safe and healthy. Clare was on the road to healing and she didn't get an infection luckily. I just did what I could to hold us all together.

The midwife instructed Emily to stay in bed for the next several days, then move to the couch for a few days after that. Emily felt so good after giving birth that this wasn't what she wanted. She asked me to help her transition from the spare room, where my son was born, to our master bedroom. This is where I had put the baby's crib just the day before and Emily wanted to stay in there. I asked her if she was ready to walk that far and sure enough, she was.

Carrying my son to his new room for the first time was a great feeling. Emily was leaning on my shoulder as she felt like her insides may fall out at any moment. She had no pain; it was just a jelly like feeling and it felt as though it was all falling.

After the long walk, Emily went potty one last time, before I brought her a stool for when she would get into bed. This is where she felt the most comfortable and wanted to be. I had changed out the linens before bringing her in here so that she had a nice fresh bed to lay in.

Laying my son in his new bed for the first time was pretty gratifying. He had slept there for 10 months inside of his mom and now he was laying in it on his own. Emily had to have a shower before getting into the bed, I made a pillow fort around my son so that he wouldn't roll away on me, as I helped her into the shower. There was blood running down her leg and she still had all of the gunk from the water birth on her skin.

I didn't join her in there, but I did wash her backside and legs and all the places that she couldn't reach. After she had her hair done and was cleaned up, I dried her off and walked her back to the bed.

I helped Emily to get settled in and I laid with them for a while. I had laundry already going and was out of chores for the time being. On high alert, it was my new job to listen for when my son would cry or fuss. When he did, I would wake mom up and help to get him nursing.

Emily would wake me up constantly throughout the night. I would not let her get out of bed or walk to the bathroom alone. It was my new job to help her change her panty liners and help clean her up after she used the bathroom. This was just like changing a diaper on my son, just at a slightly larger scale.

Each time she would get out of bed, I would change the towels under her and install fresh ones. This made for a more comfortable place for Emily to rest. This went on for days and every day that passed her bleeding was less and less. The size of her stomach was also shrinking daily.

I kept her labia clean and used honey to keep her lips from sticking together, while all the blood and gunk was still coming out of her. This worked great and she had looked brand new before the first week had even ended.

I can't stress enough that Emily wanted to get up and just do everything. It was my job to beat her to it and have it done in advance so that she couldn't. Emily was just like new after the first week.

Another thing that was imperative, was keeping Emily well fed and to make her drink plenty of water. Her lips were still chapped from the dehydration and it could have affected her breast feeding.

With Clare, and the cesarian, it took over three months for her to heal. This truly affected her breast feeding and the affection that was offered between mother and daughter. The bond was never made from the beginning and this was proven to be a negative thing in the following years.

Emily's milk was starting to come in on day four, but the baby was pretty hungry and the colostrum wasn't satisfying him. This led us to many hours of Emily and I trying to calm him down as he was hungry. By day four when the milk finally came in, boy did it start coming.

Emily was a milk factory and it was leaking everywhere. Before we started to catch it in a container it would soak the bed. Even Emily's shirts would have to be changed all day and night long.

My son was drinking like crazy; she was just producing more than he needed. This went on for the next several days until my son learned to fill his belly and he would sleep better.

Toward the end of the first week, he had the nipples figured out pretty good. Emily figured out what positions worked best to get him the most milk the easiest. Their bond is phenomenal and they are inseparable now.

Chapter 18
Dad And Baby

This was my time to get to know my new baby. I never found an excuse not to pick him up, or hold him when he was crying. I just jumped right in there and took over when needed.

I felt like it was a pleasure to me that I was able to change his first 5 diapers, before Emily even had the opportunity to change one. Let me tell you, she really missed out here. In the first 24 hours he let out what would be more poop than any baby should! It was the black tar meconium. Now, I didn't mind that so much, but he did it two days in a row!

It was my job to do the laundry, and we opted for cloth diapers. This meant that the diapers went right into the trash. I've seen a lot of things living on a farm, but what comes out of these kids is something else. I would have just burned the diapers if I could have. It was something that I will never forget, especially the way the stuff sticks to the baby. It's a miracle that it wasn't too thick to come out in the first place.

After I got through that faze, it was pretty easy from there. He had mostly just urine diapers and they are pretty easy on the washer.

Laying and watching my son sleep was also something that I enjoyed. When he would make his cheeks swell up as he smiled, I often wondered what he was dreaming about. He did need a boundary though, I didn't realize that newborns could crawl or roll over yet, well this one did. Leaving him unattended was not something I could do, so I would just take him with me on my endeavors.

Just a few hours after he was born, we walked outside into the sun and he loved it. The warmth that hit his reddish white skin seemed to soothe him. I figured if any light was safe for him to be under, it was God's light. We didn't stay out there very long, just long enough for Emily to miss him. He was even able to see the farm animals running around. This was a sneak peek into his new future and he was only hours old.

Our first shower together was pretty great also. After rubbing in the vernix that he was born with, I let him absorb it for two days. It was on his third day of life that he would have his first shower with dad. His belly button was getting pretty smelly and he needed to have any residuals of that black tar poop removed.

His first bath and it was with his dad, that's one he won't tell his friends when he grows up, I'm sure. But just in case, Emily took some pictures and he seems to like the water.

Bonding with your children is a huge part of fatherhood. I would recommend to anyone that has the chance to do it, you should take advantage of every moment you can. I even enjoy when my son is getting a diaper change and he pees across the room. It makes me kind of smile that in some way he is just showing off to me.

The whole process of At Home Delivery is something that I would encourage people to do. It's been so long since I've had a child, that it's like starting from scratch all over again. While I have the memories of the worst-case scenario; the at home experience really is the best-case scenario.

From me, the dad's point of view, there is no easy part of home birth. It takes planning, hard work and endurance. If you are willing to give it your all, you will be liberated by the results in the end. There is no better feeling as a dad, than to tell my friends and family that we had our son in our tub at home. They don't get it, they really don't. Since you are reading this book, you get it, I know you do!

Chapter 19

Finish Line

Barely twenty-four hours ago, Emily made the biggest choice of her life. Push through the pain and the tears and hold onto the one choice she would never regret. The howling that I can still hear coming from the walls of our old farm house, hasn't subsided yet. It seemed to still over power the relaxing instrumental music that I had turned on over forty-eight hours ago.

Was she really still moaning and in pain? No, it was just that I could still feel her pain inside of me. Pushing on her back for over twelve hours with only thirty seconds to a one-minute break in between, there is a connection made between Mom, Dad and Baby that I can't explain.

It's a feeling that you know the baby is safe. If he wasn't, he would somehow tell you. The other feeling is that mom no longer has to speak to you, for you to know what she wants or needs. It's these connections that will now be the new language that your body speaks without even saying a word.

What have I learned out of this experience? No matter how much you love someone and no matter the reason that you wanted to bring this precious little soul to life; the pain that Emily went through is something that I never want to hear or feel her go through again.

It is now a week later and when I close my eyes, I can still see that look on her face, when she was almost defeated. It wasn't that she couldn't do it, she was doing it for thirty-five hours. Emily is as strong as any other woman giving birth.

Emily was already there; she was giving birth at the point that we agreed to call in for backup. This wasn't a decision that I made for her; this was a decision we had made together. Going into this pregnancy we made some rules. The rules were simple. We would agree on the matter at hand at the time and both make our decisions.

Well, Emily knows that I will honor her wishes, no matter if she makes the right choices or the wrong ones. There is always going to be a discussion about it first. If she can't make her own decision, then I will intervein.

Emily made the right decision the morning my son was already crowning and I agreed with her. It was time to call in for support. We had the support system just down the road. Emily just had to prove to herself that she could take on the task of being a mother on her own.

By being a mother, it was in her DNA to deliver this baby on her own. Her body was telling her it was time, as her contractions were full term now. She was in transition by this point and there was no taking a break. That wasn't in the rule book. Yet another aspect to this, the baby was also going to decide when it was time to leave Emily's birth canal and become a new resident outside of the womb.

Was I ever scared at any time that there could be something wrong? Or that there could be another reason her moans were so intense? I was not scared. Emily needed me more than she needed anything in this world, throughout this whole process. Was I anxious? Yes, I was very anxious. Who doesn't want to see what their new child is going to look like, how his voice will sound, or how much the child will love me?

The short version of my experience is this. You better get as much sleep as you can, before the baby comes. I was expecting the baby two weeks from now, not today. Have your house in order, well before the due date. When you think that you have prepared for everything that you are about to encounter, you have forgotten a few things for sure.

Keep your grocery store trips up to date. Our refrigerator was about empty when baby decided that he wanted to come. There was no way I was going to leave Emily to go buy groceries after her water broke. The thought that ran through my mind was I would run out and miss the whole delivery.

I'm just glad that we had enough veggies left to make a pot of soup. *Pro-Tip make a giant pot of soup as soon as this whole endeavor begins.* It can just sit on the stove. Every time you pass by it, you get to take a spoonful before you're off to the next task that you will have to accomplish. Making full meals are now a thing of the past for a few days. Secondly, make her something that can deliver energy when she is getting run down. As I was making the soup, I boiled a few sweet potatoes, and added brown sugar and salt to them. This turned out to be her go to, over the soup. The soup was my go-to though.

Prepare for the unexpected. Like the fact that you will have to take over every detail that mom used to handle and I mean every detail. Once the labor starts, you can forget about leaving her side. She probably won't let you. If you're lucky enough to get a few minutes, it really won't be a few minutes. It will only be one minute at a time.

Buy a lot of extra towels! As hard as it was trying to keep up with two dogs barking, there is no time for laundry. With all of Emily's trips in and out of the shower and tub, well there isn't a lot of time to get all the wet towels dried. You will be thanking yourself if you have a pile of dry ones ready to go.

The biggest and most impactful thing that I've learned from Emily delivering our son at home is: she is a very tough person. When it comes to her protecting her child, it started way before he was ever born. Emily built this whole plan with her body to protect him from the time he was conceived. The moment she knew she was pregnant, when I saw her first tear run down her cheek, she was a changed woman.

Her whole life was different from that day forward. It was no longer about the way that she took care of herself anymore. It was now about how she took care of the little life that just decided that it would change her life for the better. There was no turning back from that day forward. Emily is no longer just my wife. She is now my Son's Mom.

Best Wishes,

Kennedy Wolf

About The Author

To say that I am an author are words that I would have never thought could come from my sun chapped lips. First, I am "DAD" then my second role as a full-time farmer comes into play.

Just like my family, the animals on the farm depend on me daily. From hauling hay to the cows in the pasture, to feeding the chickens their organic feed so they will make the best quality eggs on this earth.

Without my family our old farm is just pastures and barns that make the day pass by. But with them it's an adventure every day from the time the sun comes up until the barn doors are closed at dusk.

My son has added a new addition to carry on for me as I get older one day. I owe it all to my wife for making me want to start back over when I thought that it could have been too late.

I am thankful for the gifts that are and the ones that show up in my life what seems like every day. I don't ask for much in return, just that my family is safe and healthy.

Thank You for taking an interest in my life. *Kennedy*